natural healing for
ANIMALS

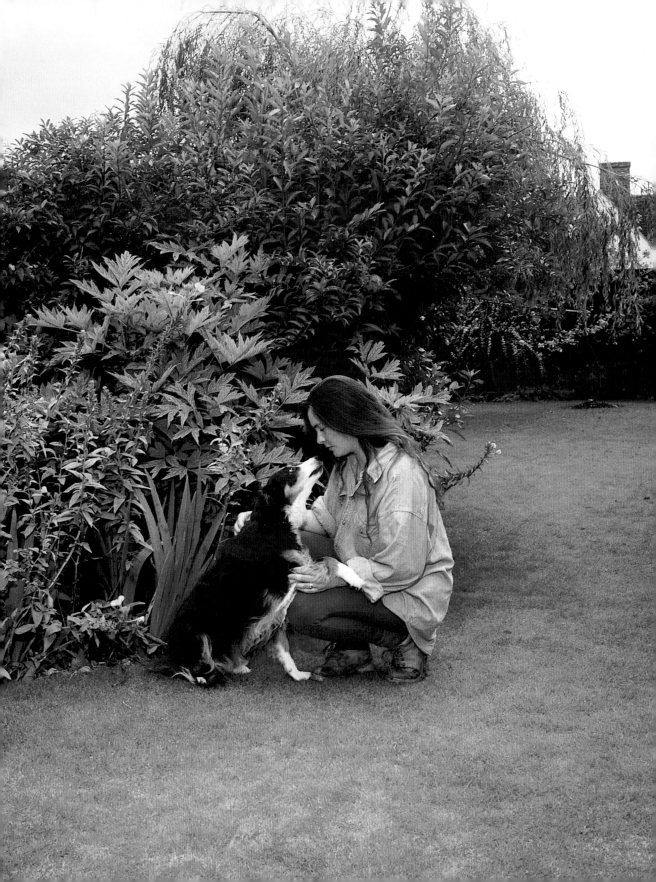

natural healing for
ANIMALS
using energy therapy at home

Clare Wilde

Kyle Cathie Limited

Thanks to animals

First published in Great Britain in 2000 by Kyle Cathie Limited
122 Arlington Road, London NW1 7HP
1 3 5 7 9 10 8 6 4 2

ISBN 1 85626 3541 360 6

Text © 2000 Clare Wilde
Special photography © 2000 Savitri Books Ltd
Also see picture acknowledgements on page 159
Design: Geoff Hayes
Editor: Lesley Gowers
Special photography: Curtis Lane & Company
Trevor Meeks

AUTHOR'S ACKNOWLEDGEMENTS

To my parents. You have both given me so much more than you will ever know. To my husband, who carries the kit as I climb mountains, watches me wave from the top, listens as I describe the view and takes a few deep breaths as I glimpse another peak to scale. To my dear friend Linda and the people who shape my life. Your influences are profoundly valuable.

To all the people and animals who I am privileged to help to learn about healing – I am honoured to be part of your lives and witness to your processes. To the people I work with on books, magazines, lectures, workshops, and in each and every thing I do – who fix my car, photocopy my notes, sell me food and make it possible for me to get through every day. You affect thousands of lives!

To the animals in my life; my guardian Pip, my wizard Dill, the gracious and beautiful April Airs, Violet the brave, the sublime Ace of Hearts and the magnificent, mighty Mole. You are each a unique source of serendipity. Thank you for coming into my life and so selflessly guiding me as I walk my path.

Clare Wilde can be contacted by E-Mail on Clare@naturalhealing.co.uk

IMPORTANT: The information given here is not intended as a substitute for veterinary advice or treatment. It is illegal for anyone other than a veterinary surgeon to diagnose, prescribe for or treat an animal. By law, the veterinary surgeon that normally treats an animal should be informed about any kind of complementary therapy that you intend to give your pet. Anyone giving therapy to an animal belonging to someone else should always make sure that they are adequately insured.

CONTENTS

INTRODUCTION

The main purpose of this book is to show how all of us can learn to help heal our pets. Much of what is written here is based on the material I teach in my workshops, where people learn how to work with healing energy to encourage their physical and behavioural conditions to heal. I would find it hard to pinpoint a single cat, dog or horse that has prompted me to write this book – it's more about the people who love those animals. Everyone I have known who has learned about healing has been thrilled to be able to do something positive to help his or her own pet. So, I felt it was time that everyone should be aware of how easy it is to learn to heal, and that all of us – yes, even you – can learn to do this quickly and simply. So many people are put off healing because they think you need to be special, gifted or just strange to be able to do it – but that isn't the case. The people who learn to do healing come from all walks of life – housewives, schoolchildren, builders, computer software engineers, and office workers – just ordinary people, with ordinary pets who need a little extra help.

Today, more of us than ever before are interested in finding natural ways to keep our animals healthy. Often, we are more concerned about caring for our animals than we are about our own wellbeing! After all, the pets who share our lives rely on us to care for them, and in return we gain the endless pleasure of their company. As we discover the limitations of the conventional medicine that is available to humans and animals, the search is on for new ways to take care of the whole individual – whatever its species! This is why I believe animals can be our teachers. Very often, they lead us on a voyage of discovery that we would never have embarked on without them – in this case, the discovery of ways to promote natural healing.

The concept of animals as our teachers is not one that is widely acknowledged in western society. In other cultures various animals are still considered sacred, as guardians and keepers of wisdom, but until very recently in the west man didn't think he had much to learn from his animals. Now, however, we are more open to trying to understand them, instead of merely finding ways to make them do as we please. In this way, animals have led and encouraged a shift in our efforts to

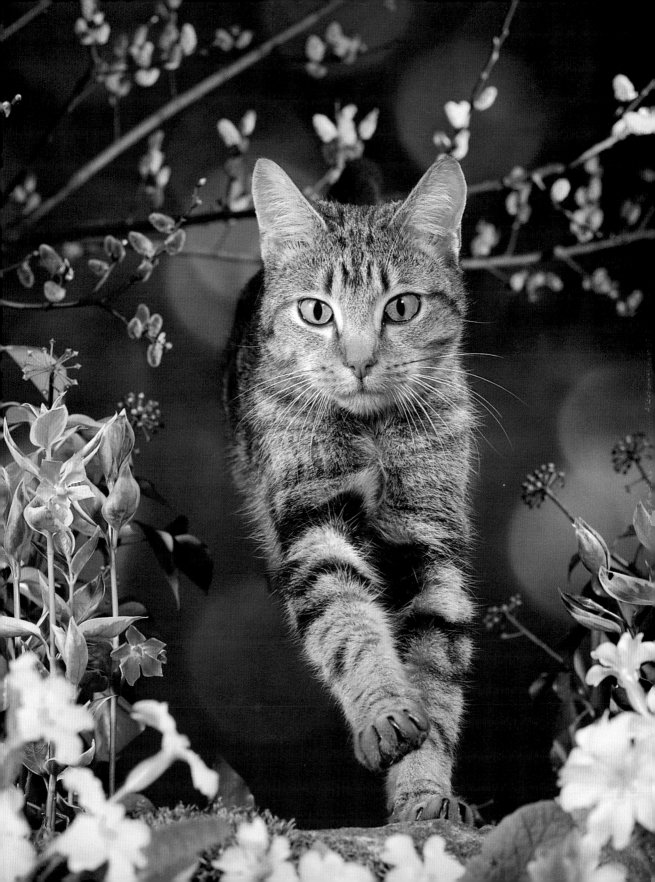

Sparkle is a nine-year-old brown and white mare – the hairy, quiet kind you tend to think of as a traveller's pony. She was doing very well at Pony Club activities with her thirteen-year-old rider, Thomas, and loved jumping and cross-country events. One August, Sparkle began to resist being mounted and then to go slightly lame; she started losing weight and became quite depressed. She was diagnosed as having a degenerative disease which affected virtually every joint of her body, and she progressively found it more and more difficult merely to stand up comfortably. To take the weight off her painful joints she would lean on the back wall of her stable. Her vets recommended that she be put to sleep, but her owner, Alison, wanted to try a different approach before she gave up on the mare.

I started treating Sparkle the following March, on alternate weeks. By May she was sound and could be ridden again, in walk at a steady pace. By July, she was flying about the countryside, putting in the odd buck and her owner asked me if I couldn't do something to reduce her energy levels! Alison attended one of my healing workshops in order to learn to treat Sparkle herself.

During the time I treated Sparkle, I also worked on the family's pet dog Teddy, who used to hang around outside the stable while I worked on the horse. Teddy, a Yorkshire terrier, suffered from mobility problems with his hind legs and had had two hip operations. The first time we met, he could only cope with a minute or two of healing but soon, he would run up to me and 'ask' for treatment. The last time I worked on him he simply rolled over and lay on his back for his healing session.

understand not just them, but each other. Thanks to our animals, the voyage of discovery we're on is taking us into new and uncharted waters and I, for one, feel privileged to be part of the adventure.

IMPROVING UPON NATURE?

There is nothing new about natural healthcare – after all, until conventional medicine became the norm that's all there was! The industrial revolution brought with it a passion for finding out what man could make, convinced that he could improve on nature. Where medicine is concerned this has often been true: many synthetic drugs act quickly and effectively to stamp out diseases that used to be the scourge of humans and animals. Vaccines now offer effective protection against many deadly diseases. Surgical procedures have improved dramatically, allowing medical and veterinary surgeons to save many more lives. But there are many conditions that do not respond well to orthodox medicine and it would take a brave individual to say that any one approach holds the ultimate answer, but in recent decades this is what many have come to believe – and old ways have been lost in favour of new ideas.

AN ALTERNATIVE TO TRADITION

The return to natural methods of healthcare has been dubbed the 'complementary', or 'alternative' approach. Many of the older generation, however, including those people from whom I have learned so much about healing, remember a time when the modern, synthetic drugs and invasive surgical procedures were the 'alternative'! Those who are exploring the 'alternatives' are seeking a way to treat the whole being, instead of working within the confines of a narrow, symptomatic approach to healthcare. In other words, it's all very well putting a plaster on a cut or giving antibiotics to fight an infection, but it is widely accepted that there is far more to disease than meets the eye. Though modern drugs have a fast, direct action on the body, they can also produce side-effects that are, at best, unwanted, and at worst, can trigger further ill health. For example, I have seen cases where antibiotics prescribed for, say, an infected wound on a cat's paw or a tear in a dog's ear, have depleted the animal's natural bacterial balance to the point where it suffers digestive difficulties as a result. Drugs that are safe and well tested are still the occasional cause of allergic reactions in some animals, and the over-use of substances like penicillin has led to a situation in which the organisms they seek to destroy, merely adapt to overcome the drug's action.

The old adage, 'a healthy mind equals a healthy body', applies not just to us, but to our animals as well. Modern medicine has one primary failing, in that it addresses only the body and not the mind. The majority of negative physical conditions have a root in mental or emotional trauma – it has been widely proven that when the mind is under stress, the immune system is suppressed, so rendering the body more susceptible to illness. Dogs and cats who are stressed or depressed, as a result, say, of being in a rescue centre, often fall prey to infections when they move to a new home, due to this very mechanism. So it's all very well relieving a set of symptoms – but what if the symptoms keep returning because the root cause of the issue has not been dealt with?

Complementary methods work to address the various factors involved in ill health, be it physical or mental, because they can influence the whole individual – in other words, they work holistically. Such methods may well take longer to produce the desired effect, because they are working to encourage the body's natural healing mechanisms – but at the same time, the unwanted side-effects are usually minimal, or non-existent. I don't propose to set complementary and traditional approaches against each other – far from it. I believe that both should exist side by side, learn from each other and acknowledge their own limitations. The idea that a single system holds all the answers is simply unrealistic, and it comes down to the way we have learned to perceive the options available to us. It's a little like the British driving on the left – it's not the only way, it's how things are at present! So, for a vet to describe an animal's condition as 'incurable' doesn't necessarily mean that it is the end of the road – simply that the conventional approach has nothing more to offer.

Many of the old remedies, such as medicinal herbs, were and still are used in a symptomatic way to treat illness, but natural herbs don't have the side-effects that so many synthetics do. Nature itself is well balanced, yet when a useful plant compound is singled out, isolating it from all the other compounds within the plant, and synthetically manufactured, the synthetic version can cause unwanted side-effects. Years ago, before so many valuable plants were considered weeds and before we all lived in tiny spaces in big towns and cities, herbs grew naturally all around us. The animals that shared our lives would thus have had access to a range of natural medicines and could select their own plant

'... to describe an animal's condition as "incurable" doesn't necessarily mean that it is the end of the road – simply that the conventional approach has nothing more to offer.'

remedies to help heal themselves. How many dog or cat owners have seen their pets happily munching away at a patch of what appeared to be weeds, but which in all likelihood are plants with medicinal properties? This behaviour is instinctive to any animal who comes across a plant that it recognizes it 'needs' – a bit like having a food craving!

NO ADDED INGREDIENTS

One of the purest, most natural and ancient methods of healthcare, however, requires no ingredients or tools and certainly has no unwanted side-effects. Since time immemorial, the laying-on of hands has been the normal and accepted way of projecting energy to the bodies of the ailing, to encourage healing. Communities throughout the world have their healers, whether that person is a religious figure or a witch. This is where our ideas spring from about who healers are – and why people feel that, unless they are religious, or a witch, healing is not something they can do. In some societies, such as native American Indians, Aborigines and in some eastern countries, healers are still the norm, and it is considered essential to consult them whenever disease strikes. However, in the west, the practice of healing with energy has been so completely lost that this kind of work is often thought of today as a little odd.

There's nothing strange about healing. If you think for a moment about your most basic reactions to pain or discomfort, you will realize that using your hands is natural. When a child comes seeking comfort for a grazed knee, any mother's automatic reaction is to rub or kiss it better. When our pets come to us hurt, unwell or in pain, the first thing we want to do is hold them. Using our hands is normal and, in fact, far more valuable than most of us realize.

IF ONLY THEY COULD TALK

You only have to watch animals together to see how powerful and important touch is to them. Whatever they do, body language and touch form an essential part of the way they communicate with each other. This is partly because animals use their senses quite differently to the way we do, and they experience the information they receive from their environments in substantially different ways

Herbal remedies can be fed in small doses to animals or used externally to help heal a variety of ailments. Camomile *Chamaemelum nobile*, shown below in its fresh and dried state, can be used as it is or decocted. It is calming to the nerves if taken internally and, if applied externally, will soothe the skin and encourage healing.

from humans. Our cats are often quiet, but use their bodies to communicate – by rubbing against us, rolling over to play, using their paws or heads to touch us, and even 'voting with their feet' – arching their backs and spitting when they're feeling angry or threatened. Dogs, though generally noisier, are more mobile – running to us and jumping up in greeting, climbing to sit on our laps, pushing against each other, and us as they play.

So, one of the main ways we can communicate with our pets, in the absence of understanding their vocal sounds, is with our bodies and through touch. Any animal trainer will tell you that body language is vital to communication and understanding. If you spend any amount of time with animals you cannot resist but touch or stroke them – it's instinctive. For most animals, being stroked by our hand is reminiscent of the licking and grooming they received from their mother when they were young, and it produces pleasant sensations of comfort and safety. This is ideal for both our animals and us – we want our pets to enjoy our company! So it's easy to see that touch can be used as a form of inter-species communication.

A healthy dog has a natural exuberance and zest for life. Activity is a dog's way of expressing his wellbeing.

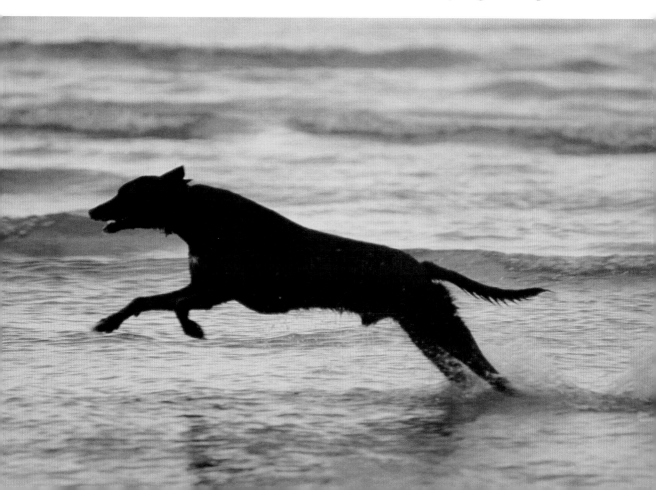

As humans, our conditioning has led us to rely heavily on a limited range of senses – mostly sight and sound. Our ways of communicating with each other cater to these senses and we tend to forget about touch and using our bodies in all but the most intimate encounters! As a result, we vastly under-use touch as a means of communication, and have forgotten how valuable it can be for exchanging information. For example, think about how you learned many of the important lessons in your life – that a match will burn you, or a nettle will sting you – through touch! The amount of information that we learn about our environment through our skin is enormous, so simple contact is far more valuable than we tend to think.

One of the most important ways that you can learn to use your hands to help your pet is to learn to exchange energy with them through touch – the laying-on of hands.

As I have said, anyone can learn healing, either through practice alone at home, or by attending a workshop, which usually just takes a single day. There are many forms of healing with energy that you can learn – from faith and spiritual healing, to those which require no faith (or spirits), such as Reiki (ray-key), Therapeutic Touch, and many more. Healing energy helps to boost the body's natural healing processes and, because information is stored in the brain, it can help to heal mental issues, too. Sparkle's owner Alison (mentioned in the case study on page 8), for example, feels much happier now that she can work to help maintain her horse's health and wellbeing without having to call in an expert to deal with routine complaints.

'... anyone can learn healing, either through practice alone at home, or by attending a workshop, which usually just takes a single day.'

ENERGY MEDICINE

In the same way that our animals, who are far closer to nature and far more instinctive than we are, sense their worlds in a different way than we do, it is possible that when man himself lived more closely to nature, his senses were sharper, too. We may have perceived our environments with an emphasis on totally different senses than those we focus on today. Now we are dulled by the constant barrage of noise and colour that comes with the modern environment. Today, if we encounter something a little odd, unexplainable, or that deviates from the 'norm', we tend to brush it aside and dismiss it, or at best, think it strange. I was lucky enough to be brought up in an environment where nothing was considered odd – whatever we experienced was something to be explored. Thus I had no limitations imposed upon my thinking. I had no idea this wasn't true for everyone, until I received feedback from a magazine article I wrote in my twenties, about how people should 'touch' their animals to help them relax or sleep. At first, the concept of working with energy does seem strange to many people – 'If I can't see it, how do I know it's real?' Well, is gravity real? – and can you *see* that?

Perhaps once, we were more able to sense the energy of the earth and our natural surroundings. Maybe this is why man settled in places which 'felt good' to him – where crops and animals thrived on the richness of the earth. Perhaps then, our sensitivity and awareness enabled us all to use our hands to project energy to help heal the bodies of sick humans and animals alike. For example – what's the first thing you do if you bang your head? Most people (after they have cursed!) will clasp their hands over the injury. Unless you work with healing energy, logically there is nothing you can achieve by doing it – but we all do it, nonetheless. Perhaps this instinctive reaction is a legacy from a time when we were all working with energy.

Placing the hands on the body to project energy is a way of recharging or replenishing the body's energy. The energy we learn to 'tune into' for healing can be thought of as similar to gravity – as a force. It's all around you, and using it helps you to feel more energetic yourself – it's a myth that healers should get tired. Some people can project energy instinctively, others learn to do it; some discover their ability suddenly, others acquire it through training. As our return to natural methods of healthcare gathers speed, energy healing has never been more acceptable and the opportunities for learning it have never been more available. Everyone can learn this simple but powerful technique to help their animals, and themselves, to heal safely and naturally.

ALL ABOUT ENERGY

THE BREATH OF LIFE

We all know what it feels like to be tired, and we all know how it feels to be full of energy. Few of us, however, stop to question where our energy comes from and what we mean when we talk about 'recharging our batteries'. Many people's best guess is that our energy comes from food, or sunlight, or air, or a combination of all three. In fact, the 'fuel' that the bodies of people and animals run on comes from a chemical reaction within the cells of the body, involving the use of carbohydrates from food, and oxygen. Neat though it is, this doesn't really go very far towards explaining what happens when that vital spark of life enters the body at the start of life, or what happens when we die. If a body is dying, it will do so regardless of whether it is fed nutrients that could enable it to continue functioning mechanically. So, what is it that comes into us at birth and leaves at death? What is that vital spark, the energy or breath of life?

Physicists now understand that all matter, everything that exists in our world, is simply a variation in form of energy. All matter is composed of atoms, and atoms in turn are composed of much smaller particles. The tiniest of these particles, when observed closely by scientists, pose quite a teaser, because when they're moving slowly enough, they are particles – but at other times, they are simply waves of energy. All 'matter', everything that we consider a solid part of our world, comes from those waves of energy. Even the atoms we're made of are never still but constantly vibrate. This vibration creates an energetic field, and so everything – a living body, a plant, a tree, or a stone on the ground (and even the ground itself) has an energy all its own.

So, the first point to understand is that everything is basically energy. The second point is that energy exists all around us. There are various kinds of energetic frequencies – some forms of which are beyond the realm of our human senses, such as waves of sound and light. The energy frequencies of TV, radio and mobile phones are way out of the range of human perception – but we know that they're there. Energies that are useful to the living body in all kinds of ways, including helping us to heal, surround us, too – and we can all learn to

Opposite. Five-month-old April Violet – my Anglo-Arab foal. Her mother, appears on page 94!

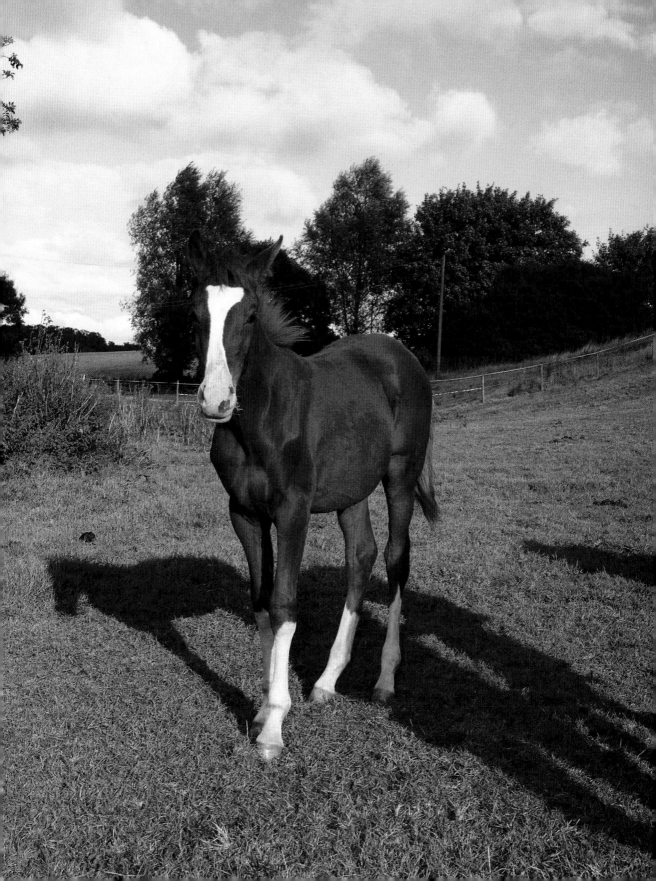

'tune in' to them. The human mind is a little like a radio – it can pick up signals that it's not normally focused on. All that is needed is a little shift of attention, practice, and/or help from another, experienced person.

The energy that exists all around us that we can use for healing is a force, such as gravity – it is real and, although it's invisible, it can be felt and measured (as an electrical charge). This energy is a constant, universal presence and living organisms – human, animal and plant – are all naturally tuned in to it to a certain extent. Our bodies draw on that energy at a constant, steady rate and it flows through the body to have a tangible benefit on health and wellbeing. In this way, the world around us can be thought of as a vast, untapped source of energy that all life – including our animals and ourselves – is a part of. Learning to 'plug in' to that energy is a great way to recharge our own bodies, and we can learn to project or 'channel' it through our hands, to other bodies to help to recharge them, too. I often tell people to think of the first 'Star Wars' film where Luke Skywalker learns from an ancient guru-teacher about 'the force'. Luke learns how to 'use the force' for all kinds of beneficial purposes. If it sounds like a coincidence, I should point out that George Lucas was inspired to write the 'Star Wars' films by the teachings of Joseph Campbell, a pioneer in understanding spirituality and the energy fields related to life!

In the normal, healthy, living body, energy (some people call it 'bioenergy') is drawn steadily in from outside, and flows through and around it to maintain wellbeing. How people understand this principle depends upon their own culture or belief system. In eastern medicine, the concept of the individual as a system of energetic pathways is familiar and well understood. The west, however, favours a more mechanical understanding of what life is and means in terms of the body as a functioning unit. Chinese medicine, for example, recognizes the physical body as having a system of pathways or tiny tubes of energy called meridians. Whenever the flow of life energy (often called Chi or Ki) is obstructed or is low, the body is more prone to illness. The meridians have been the subject of many experiments and can be identified and measured – they 'pop up' to the surface of the body at certain points. Therapies like acupuncture, acupressure, shiatsu and reflexology all work with points on the meridians to release blockages and encourage a clear flow of energy around the body, so promoting health and wellbeing. These treatments are now widely available to people and animals, but healing with energy is said to be more effective than any of these treatments, because it can so effectively address the whole system. Aside from this, animals find healing particularly pleasant as it's completely non-invasive – there is no pressure from the hands and you can even work with your hands a little way off the body.

Ayurveda, India's ancient medical system, and the Buddhist one too, work with a system of energy centres, like whirlpools, on the body, called chakras. The main chakras are located down the centre line of the body. Again, whenever these energy centres are blocked or obstructed and the flow of life-force is interrupted, the body is more prone to disease. Still other forms of western therapy, such as cranio-sacral work and cranial osteopathy, recognize the mid-line of the body as the centre of energy and life; especially the navel area, where life first comes into the embryo from the mother via the umbilical cord. When you use energy to heal, you tap into your natural process of drawing in energy from outside, but in a more accelerated way. That way, you can project the extra 'outside' energy out through your hands, and leave the resources your own body needs intact or even boosted.

As well as fuelling the living organism to maintain life and health, energy surrounds the body in a field, often called the aura. The aura is said to be where energetic disturbances first occur and, if they become compounded, are eventually manifested in the physical body. The auras of animals and children, in particular, are wide open to influences from outside. This living energy field has been photographed, using a technique called Kirlian photography, which captures the energetic imprint of the subject. Kirlian photographs have been taken not just of the living energy field of humans and animals, but also of plants, and even energy medicines such as essential oils. Many people learn to feel auras, and some can see the energy fields of not only the living, but also inanimate objects such as stones. Once you begin to realize that all matter has its own tangible energy field, it isn't so difficult to see how projections of healing energy can be absorbed not just by animals and people, but by plants and even objects such as crystals.

A FORGOTTEN ART

The fact that so many cultures recognize the body as an energy system is evidence of the way that energy is, and has always been used the world over to encourage healing. In the west, we have largely lost or forgotten the healing arts

'In the west, we have largely lost or forgotten the healing arts that, to our ancestors, were probably part of everyday life...'

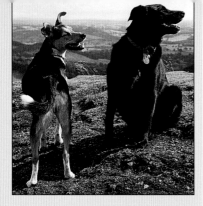

Dill breathes freely

Dill is my own dog who came from an animal shelter. As soon as he moved in with us he showed signs of kennel cough, and within forty-eight hours he was hacking away constantly. He had a high temperature, a discharge from his nose and was having difficulty breathing normally. His appetite was gone and he became very lethargic, his behaviour changing dramatically over the course of the next twenty-four hours to the point where he was a very sad little dog.

I began treating him with healing energy as often as I could, besides feeding him garlic and honey to help fight off infections and soothe his airways. He was given sticks of pinewood to chew, as the vapours are also good for a congested chest. At night, I rubbed a blend of essential oils around his collar which included eucalyptus, peppermint and lemon. This also helped to clear his nose and throat. His energy levels started to improve significantly following the treatments and he slowly began to improve. Suddenly, after four days, he perked up, started playing again and was obviously feeling much better. All symptoms of his illness were gone within a further forty-eight hours. He was young and his system rapidly developed its own immunity, enabling him to return to full health. I continue to treat him and it's hard to believe that it is the same animal. He certainly has no lack of energy now!

that, to our ancestors, were probably part of everyday life, in the same way that so many other 'natural' methods of healthcare were. Countries like China, India, and parts of Africa and Australia, for example, still retain the healing practices that have been handed down through the generations. In India and China, for example, herbalists, healers and practitioners of traditional medicine are as commonplace as general doctors in the western world. Such people live with healing as an accepted and often, essential method of bringing the body back into balance – of using energy to boost the flagging or fluctuating energy levels of the living. The bodies of people and animals are healed, and even the energy of the land itself, by religious figures such as priests, tribal leaders, witch-doctors, shaman and wise women.

The belief held by many different ancient cultures that energy 'animates' or gives life to matter and the living body is often called 'animism', from the Latin *anima*, meaning soul. Animistic beliefs are based on the idea of people, animals, rocks, trees and plants, all having a soul energy – in other words, that all matter has energy! If such ancient cultures knew all this, how come it's taken western scientists so long to agree? The derivation of the word 'animal' from *anima*, is a clear label for the physical expression of a soul, or an energetic force within a living being.

Energy, like air or water, is universal, and cannot be contained by geography or language. The way in which it is used varies little from one continent to the next – a simple laying-on of hands. This ritual has even been retained in cultures who have lost the healing arts in something of a 'race memory' – automatically placing our hands over an injury – which is a quirk of human behaviour which has no basis in logic – unless you're doing healing!

OUR COMPANION ANIMALS

One of the more natural and ancient habits that the western world has retained is that of living closely with animals as companions. Humans the world over esteem and value animals, often in very different ways. In the west, our respect for individual animals often depends upon their breeding and financial value. In other cultures, however, status is given to species of animal as powerful forms of the raw energy in nature (the 'animal' as the soul or *anima* of nature). People in ancient cultures such as the native American Indians, are even given names derived from animals as totems to give them strength, protection and guidance.

In the west, the last echoes of this tradition were finally abolished as recently as two centuries ago as witch-hunts took their toll. The wise men and women who worked with nature (especially with herbs) and had companion animals as guides, were put to death, fled to avoid persecution, or were forced to adopt more 'normal' lives. One of the criteria for being a witch was to live in close company with an animal, and the degree of the witches' powers were often judged according to the names, and species, of their 'familiars'. For example, the name 'Grizzle' for a cat, meant its owner was definitely a witch – and if the cat was black, then it was probably an emissary of the devil, so the owner must therefore be the worst kind of witch! In the area where I live, witch-hunts were rife, and well known wise women were imprisoned and killed just for being able to influence animals' behaviour. These attempts to stamp out healing and close human/animal relations sealed in many minds the idea that healing arts, using herbs and other natural medicines, were definitely to be avoided. This became so well imprinted on the popular psyche that many people still view natural medicine with a dose of suspicion.

A hissing, angry cat can be quite frightening. Perhaps for this reason, cats were often associated with witches, black cats in particular were well-known 'witches' familiars', yet for some people seeing a black cat meant good luck.

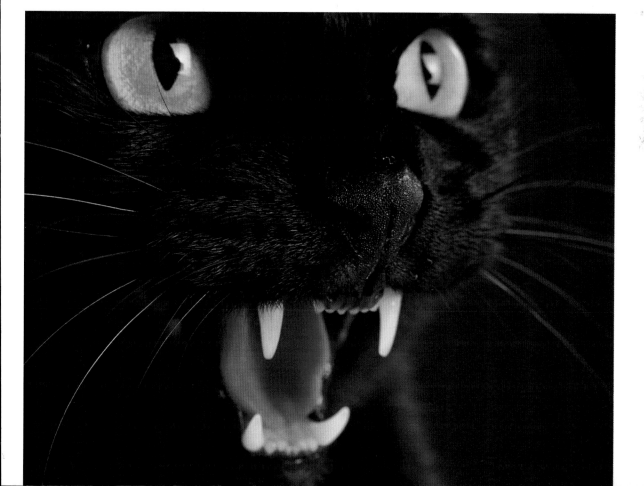

UN-COMMON SENSES

Since those times, our attentions have been focused well and truly on what is acceptable and normal to society. Our enthusiasm for forgetting natural methods of healthcare has resulted in us denying anything 'out of the ordinary' that we experience, like knowing who is on the telephone before we pick it up. At best we dismiss such happenings as coincidence, and at worst, we have learned to fear that our revelations might not be quite acceptable to everyone else! It's safer, and more acceptable, for us to believe only what we can see, and not to 'feel' anything untoward. So, we exist in a state of very low awareness, generally focusing only on what we choose to look at (often for amusement or to perform a task as part of our work), or listen to. This is why accidents can happen so easily in the home and other places that we perceive to be so safe – because we aren't alert to our surroundings. If you take away the noise, colour and distraction and simply remain aware of your environment, ideally out in the open countryside, your senses will begin to focus on other information – which can give us a little insight into how life feels for our animals.

People who live with animals are often concerned with how their pets feel – happy or unhappy, playful or tired, hungry or sleepy – and spend a lot of time observing them closely. It is easy to see that many of our animals know when, for example, bad weather is coming, or even what kind of mood their owners are in. How many humans have such acute perception, or would admit to it if they had? As Leslie Kenton, the well-known writer, says, 'animals simply sense, whereas humans sense that they sense'. It's that space which gives our intellect time to question what we're sensing – 'did I imagine that?' But if you just stop to think, for a moment – how many of you know what your animals need or want simply by they way they look or sit? How many of you have known exactly what someone was about to say to you? There is much more to life than meets the eye.

THE LANGUAGE OF ENERGY

Thinking in this way begins to open our minds to the idea that humans can and do have a wider range of untapped perceptive senses. For example, while it can be limiting, the language we use is in fact a very clear key to some of our more abstract perceptions. Much of our language is simply our brain's attempt to process the information it receives from the environment. There are all kinds of expressions we use to convey feelings that we haven't felt with our bodies. When you meet someone and talk to them, you might use expressions like 'I felt so comfortable with him'; 'We were really sparking off each other'; or 'She was really grating on me'. Generally there have been no sparks, no one has grated anybody else and largely, given the accepted social behaviour surrounding touch, it is highly unlikely that we have 'felt' each other at all, in a physical sense. These are all phrases for a 'feeling that someone has given us' either through their behaviour, language or how they use their own energy. Individuals who are calm, happy and vital will have an energy field that reflects the way they feel. On coming into contact with them, we experience pleasant, soothing, and often reviving sensations somewhere 'out there' and translate this mentally into a word. Individuals who are angry or stressed will have an energy field that reflects their jagged, scattered state and we can feel that in no uncertain terms. Often we will begin to protect ourselves using our bodies and voting with our feet – by walking away. Spending time with our animals, whose simple energy is so calming, is known to be highly therapeutic to humans.

Put this way, it's easy to see that most of us do 'sense' and 'feel' things in other ways than are generally accepted as standard. Simply because so much of our life is spent with a very narrow focus of attention, our perceptive senses are vastly under-used and underdeveloped. Humans have surrounded themselves with a complex game of language and protocol where body language is ignored or purposely masked to serve our own ends. We can communicate by words alone – for example, by letter or e-mail, and hold a pretty good written 'conversation' without even needing to physically see the other person!

ANIMAL MAGIC

There are, however, more and more of us today who have the freedom and the interest to explore our perceptive feelings and are looking beyond what meets the eye. We are beginning to open ourselves to the world around us again. When people learn to work with energy and experience the effects it can have on their animals (and indeed, witness the profound reactions that animals can have to a healing treatment), any scepticism is dissolved and arguments about it being 'all in the mind' are quickly forgotten. After all, animals merely exist and react – they just 'sense' – they don't have to think about whether or not to respond to what they feel, they just do.

Because animals work on a far less intellectually messy and more instinctive level than humans do, their experience of 'feeling' or 'sensing' is clearer, sharper and not obscured by mental chatter – 'Is this normal? Did I feel that?' They can sense our anger or happiness, and even health and sickness, on a very basic level. Perhaps this is because their perceptive senses are more acute than our own, dulled repertoire of 'feelings'. The animals we share our lives with are likely to have a far more complete 'energy picture' than we do, of the environments in which they live as well as the other animals and objects they encounter in daily life. To start with, their senses can operate on a different range to ours – they can hear noises that we can't! Aside from this, they are far more aware of body language and movement generally than we are, as this is a major factor in determining whether another animal is friend or foe.

It may well be that this acute perception of movement and energy is what 'draws' animals to certain people and leads them to avoid others – simply according to how each individual 'feels' to them. I have clients who are shocked when their pet cat or dog would much rather stay with me than go to them after a healing treatment. There are all kinds of remarkable stories from modern newspapers back through the legends and fables of time, about how various animals have 'known' things in some kind of super-sensitive way. These vary from dolphins rescuing a drowning sailor or child, horses carrying a wounded soldier gently and safely home from the battlefield, cats returning to a home they have moved away from – often covering vast distances, to dogs alerting other people to help their endangered owners (what else was 'Lassie' based on?).

Passionflower *(Passiflora incarnata)* is used for its calming and soothing properties. It is suitable for people and animals. The stem and leaves are used when dried.

Because animals react so instinctively to the information they receive from their environment, it is easy to see how the body operates simply as a manifestation of what's going on in the mind. If the information the brain receives is processed in such a way as to require and produce a response, the impulses within the brain send messages to the cells that, for example, can produce a movement in a muscle. The simplest way to translate this into everyday life is to look at the way that teaching an animal a word-command can produce certain types of behaviour – for example 'no', 'sit', and of course, 'dinner'! This is as a result of stimulus-response conditioning and the way that the brain processes information – in through the body to the brain, and then out again through the body. Of course, it is impossible to make a distinction between mind and body because the individual being is a whole – but in terms of healing, dis-ease (negative physical condition) is often split into a physical or emotional condition. In fact, we are simply dealing with levels of energetic disturbance. One neat way to understand the inextricable connection between mind and body is to look at the way that the brain affects physical behaviour, and vice versa.

BODY, BRAIN AND BEHAVIOUR

The cells that make up the living body serve all kinds of purposes and come in all shapes and sizes. Each kind of cell has a different name according to the purpose it serves – or the job it does. Receptor cells, as the name suggests, are involved in receiving information from the environment and are found all over the body – for example, in the eyes, ears and skin. So, receptors can be thought of as sense cells, because they are involved in processing information from the environment through what we call the 'senses'. Energy that sense cells receive is sent as an impulse, via the nerve cells, to the brain. The receptor cells found in the skin are sensitive to stimuli such as touch. If you stop to consider the size of the skin as an organ in relation to the rest of the body, and the number of sense cells within the skin, you can see that the volume of information received this way is potentially enormous.

The brain is made up of clumps of nerve-endings including, of course, the endings of the nerve cells that transmit messages from the sense cells to the brain. The brain processes and stores the information received from these nerve cells. It also signals impulses to the nerve cells that travel from the brain to influence physical behaviour – for example, to move a muscle. The impulses, or charge of each cell can be measured, using sensitive instruments like a voltmeter. So the mental and physical, the mind and body are a whole, and not two separate systems or entities at all. It's important to bear this in mind as you look at the causes and healing of dis-ease from a holistic viewpoint.

So, the body can be thought of in terms of energetic impulses travelling from one cell to another, carrying information and influencing behaviour. This can help us to understand how making energy available to the body can offer new information, not just on a physical level, but also in terms of the information

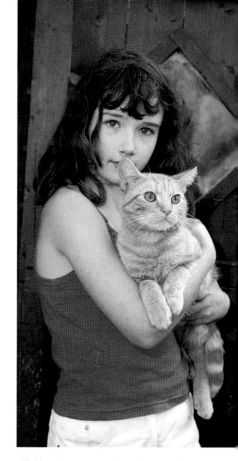

Children love an animal as their special play-mate. The simple friendship shared between child and pet is a good education for human relationships in later life.

> *'Working with energy is truly holistic... Energy therapy can heal "memory scars" or negative information held within the brain.'*

processed by the brain – in other words, on a learned, emotional or behavioural level. Such an energetic exchange also provides a means of release of information in the same way – and this is one way in which healing can be understood to take place. Because energetic exchange does not discriminate between the cells and their function, it can also be said to occur totally holistically – on every level of the individual.

THE HEALING TOUCH

In the absence of Dr Doolittle-like qualities, and without being able to experience the world in the way that our animals do, we learn to use energy to communicate with and heal our animals. Touch is obviously important to our animals for communication, and, in terms of the cells of the body, it is easy to see the vast potential for exchange of information through touch. The touch of a hand on the body can be used to calm and still, to comfort and relax, to encourage movement, to teach and even to heal.

If you learn to transmit energy to other bodies through touch, you can also facilitate healing by positively influencing the cells of the body. It doesn't matter whether the body in question is canine, feline, equine or human. By drawing in the energy that is all around us, and projecting it by laying our hands on others, we can recharge negative energy, helping to shift blockages and stimulate physical healing.

Working with energy in this way is truly holistic. As well as addressing physical symptoms, it can work to recharge and strengthen the animal's energy field, so that any disruptions are cleared before they materialize as a physical problem. Energy can also help to recharge on a basic, cellular level and thus to heal 'memory-scars' or negative information held within the brain, and the way that this learned information has come to affect behaviour. Using energy as a healing therapy is also the most accessible form of self-help there is, contrary to popular myth. It's portable, it's silent, and can be done absolutely anywhere. Anyone can learn to work with energy, and doing so raises the energy levels of the practitioner as well as the patient – nourishing the body, and leaving both feeling revitalized and refreshed.

GETTING IN TOUCH WITH ENERGY

WHO CAN DO IT?

You can. It follows that, because energy is available everywhere and to every living being, there are no boundaries regarding who can learn to work with energy to encourage healing. I believe it is true that the ability to tune into ambient energy is latent in everyone. For some people, this ability will be strong, clear and workable – all it takes to translate this into working practice is a little guidance or perhaps just patience and experience. Some people may be 'doing something' with energy and have an idea of what is going on – but need to have their suspicions reinforced or confirmed! For others, the ability is there but the confidence or self-belief in that ability is lacking and help is needed to encourage the ability to flow. For others, the way to tune into energy has been forgotten and some 'tweaking' is required in terms of training. However, there is nothing mysterious, exclusive or secret about using energy – anyone can learn to do it.

For those of you who are working naturally with energy, the first clues you will have that something is happening are likely to be the responses of those you work on. These will range from deep relaxation and drowsiness, to a feeling of invigoration following treatment. People may comment on feeling warmth or tingling, or a flowing sensation from your hands. Animals will simply respond in the most obvious way possible – by making it perfectly clear that they love what you're doing – often they will become still or sleepy as you touch them. For yourself, you might notice feelings in your palms and fingertips of warmth, pins and needles, throbbing or itching – you may even see redness in your hands as you work. Energy is naturally pulled by the body of the individuals you're working on as they need it, so you might find that certain people or animals seem to produce a strong reaction in your hands whilst others have a less dramatic effect.

Ginger's battle scars

Ginger is a big, handsome male cat who, in spite of being neutered, is the Casanova of his neighbourhood! Needless to say, this causes problems for him, particularly when new cats move in and out of the area. Ginger comes home scratched and bitten whenever he's been fighting, which means another visit to the vet to be treated for wounds and infections. Keith, his owner, learned healing to treat Ginger himself at home and help cut down the recovery time from his battle scars.

After one particularly bad fight, Ginger had his ear stitched by the vet and Keith gave him healing energy. Ginger seemed very sorry for himself after he'd been patched up. 'When we got home, I took Ginger out of his travelling basket and sat with him on my lap, stroking him and giving him healing. He stretched out on his side, and lay his head, with the stitched ear downwards, right in my palm. I knew he felt poorly, but as I held his little head, he became completely still. In that moment, I really felt that he knew I was helping him, and that he had given me his total trust. He's not really a lap cat, but he is now much more affectionate and I feel so much closer to him.' Keith now also feeds Ginger a herbal mixture, which acts as a natural antibiotic, to help deal with any infections he might sustain.

Ginger is one of many cats who are very sensitive to healing energy and who seem to seek it from their owners. They love to come and join in healing workshops. I remember once at a student's house when, as she first began to project energy from her hands, her cat sat down in front of her, and gazed right into her eyes as if to say: 'When do I get to try this out?' There was such a moment of connection that we felt the little cat knew exactly what was going on.

If you work naturally with energy, or have already undertaken some kind of formal training in healing, you will simply be able to follow the guidelines for treatment given later in this book. With practice, you will very quickly be able to treat your animals, yourself and other people as necessary. For those who have an inkling that they are using energy already but aren't quite sure, my advice would be to try some treatments, to practise and see what happens. One lady who came to me for training said that her hands tingled whenever she put them over her cat's operation scars, and that her cat fell asleep. 'Excellent,' I said, 'you're already projecting energy from your hands!' She looked absolutely amazed. 'Am I?' she asked. 'Well, that's a relief. I thought there was something wrong with me!' She had been quite worried about doing any kind of healing work on her cats at home because she just wasn't sure what she was dealing with, nor if it was OK to dabble without any supervision.

This kind of experience is typical in those who are sensitive to energy. I have met people who can naturally feel 'holes' or blockages in their pet's energy, but have had no idea how to help heal them. I have taught many students whose hands tingled or throbbed as they placed them over the sites of injuries. There are others, like me, who send animals to sleep simply by touching them, who just 'know' what is wrong, and who find that afterwards, the animals seem to recover very quickly. However, I was lucky enough never to have been worried that this was odd or unusual, so I never lacked the confidence in what I was doing. Much of the time, it's simply that – a question of confidence. With energy healing, you can never do any harm and you may well see some startling and encouraging results! The practice of tuning into healing energy is a little like flexing a muscle – the more you use it, the stronger it becomes.

HOW DO I START?

The first and easiest way to learn to feel energy with your hands is to rest them a little way above the skin of another person or animal. You can even do this by moving the palms of your own hands towards and away from each other – it might help if you rub your hands together first, which helps to sensitize them and ensures that your own energy is not stagnant, but is moving around freely. Gently and very slowly move your hands up and down, away from and towards each other or the surface of the body you're working on, until you find a height where you can feel a cushioned or magnetic feeling. You can also experience this sensation if you hold your hands a few inches apart, and ask someone else to move their hand into the space between yours, and out again. This is a great way to begin to feel the difference between someone or something else's energy field, and your own. The 'cushion' that you begin to feel is the closest and densest layer of the energy field of the person or animal you are working with. Most people start to feel these sensations if not straight away, then within a few minutes of practice.

If you're in doubt about what you feel, or feel nothing at all, then stop for a few minutes, rub your palms together again, and try moving your palms towards each other from a distance of about twelve inches (30cm) apart. It helps if you do this with your eyes closed. Move your hands very slowly, and open your eyes only when you feel the 'cushion'. You will begin to experience the energy 'cushion' between your own hands at around four to six inches (10–15cm) distance apart – it feels like a definite tingling, and slight pressure, almost as if you're holding a very soft, light fluffy ball. Some people prefer to try this exercise when they're alone, so that what other people feel or say doesn't influence them. If you don't feel something immediately, go and do something else, forget about it for a while, and then try again later. Rest assured that, with a little patience, everyone can begin to experience the feeling of their own energy and that of other people and animals with this simple method.

If you experiment, and focus as you move your hands very slowly around the body at a similar height, where you can feel the energy 'cushion', you may find that you begin to experience feelings of heat, warmth, cold, tension or weakness under your hands. Sometimes you will just stop, and then the thought pops into your head – 'hang on, something feels different there'! With practice, you can learn to translate these feelings in energy terms, and understand what is happening in the energy field of the animal or person you're working on. For example, an area that feels weak indicates a lack of energy; cold indicates a blockage; tension or a sort of bumpy feeling may be the site of a current or old injury; warmth is a healthy area; and heat is a strong energetic pull. Some people learn to see energy as a distortion around or within the body as they're working with their hands, while others visualize it in their mind's eye or hear energy as it moves. So don't be too surprised by the sensations you may experience as you start to work.

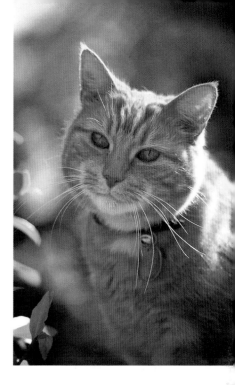

Above. Ginger – 'the Casanova of his neighbourhood' – whose story appears on the left-hand page. Below. Golden hamster. Hamsters make charming pets, but they need plenty of fun and games in their cage.

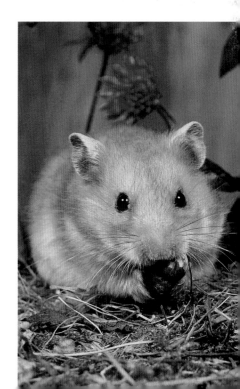

If you have a willing partner to practise on, ask this person for feedback, so that you can compare what each of you feels. A good subject is a friend or partner who, whilst not so sceptical as to be 'blocked' to what you're doing, or afraid of what they might feel, will be honest and not just say they're experiencing all kinds of sensations to keep you happy! As you gain confidence about what you feel in your hands, you will find that you begin to experience more warmth or tingling in your palms or fingertips. At the same time, you should begin to 'look for' or 'tune in' mentally to the feeling of energy coming into your body, usually through the top of your head. This is how it feels when you begin to make a connection to a much wider source of energy than your own – the energy that is available all around us. As you begin to connect to this energy, it will flow more freely through your hands to the body of the recipient. All of this takes time, focus at first, and inevitably, practice, but it is one of the key ways in which people begin to discover their own ability to draw in and project energy to the bodies of others.

You can, of course, practise all of this on your pets, but the responses you receive may be more difficult to interpret (I have given pointers about how animals are likely to react to treatment in the next chapter).

It is also important to remain objective and aware of what you are experiencing. The more practice you get, the more sensitive you will become to cues from your hands. In this way you may find that your ability to connect with healing energy is awakened simply through use alone, and without any training at all.

Though at first this work may take a little concentration, it is important to state here that in no way should it leave you feeling tired or drained. If you are tuning into and picking up ambient energy (which often feels like a slight prickling or pressure at the crown of your head), you will feel refreshed and invigorated as the energy flows through you. Practitioners of one healing art or another who claim to feel exhausted following treatments are projecting their own energy. This is unhealthy for the practitioner, who then has to resource a fresh energy supply for himself – usually, by lying down to recuperate. It is also unhealthy for the recipient of the treatment, who is receiving energy not from an abundant, fresh source, but from the body of the practitioner. This is hardly something most of us would wish for. If you feel worn out following energy work, it is advisable to stop and seek guidance or tuition, because you may be someone who is very good at the 'energy out' part, but not so good at 'energy in'!

'The more practice you get, the more sensitive you will become to cues from your hands.'

WHAT DO I GET?

Those who have hitherto had no leanings in this direction, will find that the increased sensitivity and awareness of their own bodies and minds opens up a whole new way of thinking and feeling. Often, learning to work with energy can benefit people who have long-term health or emotional problems and want to improve their energy levels and overall wellbeing. Many people find that the spin-off benefits of learning to work with energy, aside from helping to heal themselves and their own animals, might include helping a sick or elderly parent or relative, their family, and pets belonging to friends and neighbours.

The benefits of learning to work with energy are countless and it is true to say that it can bring about a profound shift in the quality of your life. Some of the tangible benefits are increased personal energy levels, the ability to relax more deeply, a sense of inner strength, clarity of mind, greater awareness and sensitivity, and the ability to self-treat whenever you so desire. Long-term, significant changes can take place in terms of one's own health. Of course, for the animals in your life, the benefits are countless and are based upon not only being able to receive treatments ad-lib for existing or newly arising conditions, but the greater benefit of receiving regular energy top-ups as a means of preventive natural healthcare. It can also strengthen and deepen the bond between you and your pet simply by allowing you to connect with him on a much deeper and more subtle level than ever before.

Keith and Ginger's experiences, related on page 26, are not isolated cases. I have heard many, many stories from people who report that, as they become more sensitive to energy and more practised at working with healing, they tend to know far more about what their pets are thinking and feeling. Sometimes this bond develops as your pet learns that he can be given some healing energy just by asking for it. For example, Ross, a Great Dane that I treated some time ago, always used to bound up to me and force himself into my hands when I arrived to treat the family's horses. Carol, his owner, could never understand why because I was there to treat her horses. However, when she learned healing herself, she found that while she was working on the horses, Ross would stand outside the stable door on his hind legs, peering in, as if to say, 'Is it my turn yet?' Remarkably, Ross actually 'swapped loyalties' from Carol's husband, Nick, to Carol – simply because he just loved getting healing from Carol!

> *'Often, learning to work with energy can benefit people who have long-term health or emotional problems and want to improve their energy levels and overall wellbeing.'*

GETTING STARTED

Keith and Carol are just ordinary people, just like all the other student healers I know. There are no qualifications needed, no special talents or preparation required before taking training in healing. The basic skills of most healing arts can be learned simply, quickly and inexpensively, often in just a day. Rest assured, if you have doubts – in all the workshops I have taught, everyone arrives secretly afraid that they're the one who won't be able to 'do it'. This never, ever happens! The mere fact that people want to learn is often enough for them to start to make the connection for themselves. It's true that working with energy may come more naturally to some than to others; and that some may struggle with the logic or explanation of how this unseen force is flowing through them. A word of comfort – after a while, you give up questioning, and simply learn to let it happen.

There are several martial arts that serve to increase your ability to draw in and project energy, such as Tai Chi and Qi Gong. In China and Japan, where these practices originated, masters of the martial arts are often considered to have the ability to use their increased energy levels to heal, due to their enhanced awareness of energy and heightened ability to project it. Whilst these techniques can undoubtedly help in terms of energy projection, however, they can involve rigorous exercise and training and in some cases, many years of work to reach the required levels of energy projection. In contrast, most healing energy therapies can be taught simply and easily.

Touch is vital to the wellbeing of cats, as indeed of all pets. Healing energy therapy can be given as often as desired and form part of the loving relationship between owner and pet. It can be done with the animal on your lap or while he relaxes on your bed, or simply when you stroke him.

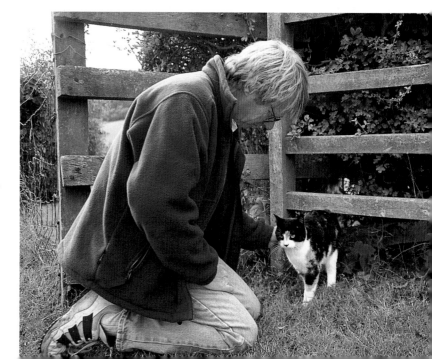

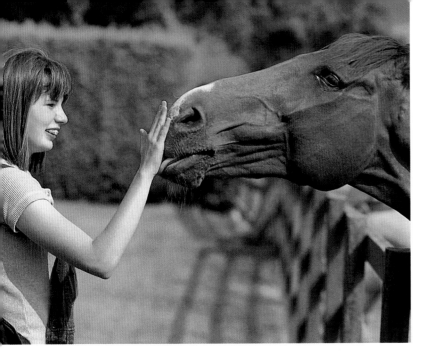

Animals are sensitive to people who work with energy and will come to nudge your hands, or otherwise 'ask' for a treatment.

With many forms of healing practice, the ability to connect to the energy you are seeking to draw in, is given by the teacher to the student, in the process known as an 'attunement' – literally, helping someone to 'tune in'. This is simply a way of reminding you how to work with energy. Some teachers describe attunements as being a way of using energy to heal the memory, and thus to revive the knowledge of how to draw in energy and use it to heal. Whilst the form of the attunements varies between one healing art and the next, and even between teachers of the same method of healing, it is interesting to note that similar processes are found in widely dissimilar cultures around the world. These include the Tibetan Buddhists (who have an empowerment ritual), the Russian orthodox church, the Aborigines and even, some might say, the modern Church of England ceremony of christening.

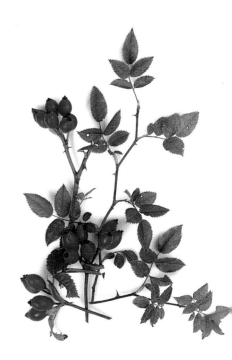

Roseships are free food and offer a natural source of many nutrients, including vitamin C.

Some of us are more naturally inclined to work with energy than are others, in the same way that some of us will find it easier to ride a bicycle or drive a car than others. However, once the basics have been established, there is rarely much to choose between the 'natural' healer and one who has been trained. Indeed, training can serve to strengthen the energies and ability of natural healers. It is true, though, that some people will find it easier to cope with working with energy than others, particularly if you begin to treat animals other than your own, or this becomes your profession. The kind of tact and empathy required to help other animals and people from all walks of life successfully on a daily basis often requires a deeper understanding of animal and human nature than can be gained on a short training course. In this respect, there is no substitute for experience.

We tend to think of the people who are most able to empathize with others or who have long-standing experience of understanding animals, as sensitive. Often this sensitivity is not innate but is learned through experience, which enables them to identify with the problems they come across. Those who have gone through serious illness, or life-changing events realize that life is for living, not for being sick, and learn to live their lives to the full. It is exactly this sort of experience that can be of great benefit in helping others to heal – people call it 'the dark night of the soul'; their own learning process whereby their understanding of life shifts dramatically. After training. many students who have experience of nursing their own animals through sickness, turn to helping animals. This is just another way in which animals act as our guides and teachers. The events and processes involved in caring for one animal can be of great benefit in caring for others in similar situations, and bring great comfort to owners who feel isolated by their pet's illness.

No amount of reading, or lessons with a teacher can be a substitute for this kind of experience. Any study you undertake or course you attend is merely the first step along your path, and the bulk of what you learn about healing will come as you gain experience through practical work, which is the best way to gain experience. Finding the confidence actually to practise and use your new-found ability, is one step that many find daunting – but once you take it there's no turning back! If you're going to work on your own pets, you can get started quietly and without too much trepidation just by going home and getting down to it – most people can't wait!

Healing is about compassion for other living beings, and it is vital to bear this in mind at all times. The principle of compassion is that your ethics and intent remain true. Although we all have to have some personal boundaries, helping others to heal, particularly animals, is about being unconditional and offering energy to the body as it needs it. This means that you don't give healing cluttered by your own desires for outcome or concerns with results. The energy comes through you, not from you, so the results or outcome are not up to you – they are up to the body of the recipient of the energy. You cannot force healing upon any animal (even if they don't know you're going to work on them). Having said this, some of the strongest healing comes from a loving heart and it is worth remembering that as you give healing, you make a deeper connection than merely that of hand on body. The body will draw only the energy it needs and therefore the agenda for change is deeply individual. I will discuss this in greater detail in Chapter 6.

MAKING THE CONNECTION

For those who are struggling to get going on their own, or who would like to undertake formal training or receive guidance from a teacher, there are various options available. In my experience there is something synchronistic about finding your teacher – often the right individual just seems to pop up, or make their presence known to you. The path you choose, and the style and manner in which you take your training, will depend largely upon how you perceive the ability to work with energy. For many people, it is easy to see it as a latent ability that is perfectly natural; we simply need 'reminding' about how to use it. For others, it may be perceived as, for example, a gift from God.

Whatever your philosophy, you will easily find someone who can tutor you. There are spiritual healers, faith healers, those who work naturally and don't question it, those who work with earth energy, and all kinds of recognized healing therapies such as Therapeutic Touch, Reiki and Seichem. Fundamentally, these forms of energy work are very similar. I learned to do Reiki to reinforce the healing I was already doing, because it is so quick and simple to pick up.

The one thing that it is vital to remember at all times is that the energy does not, and should not, come from you – you are simply the tool, or conduit for the energy. If it's your own pet that you are lucky enough to help to recover from ill health, the feeling of trust you develop in a tool like healing is enough to allay all your personal fears. Remember – healing is always worth a try – it might just be the answer you're looking for.

'Those who perceive themselves as having some kind of special 'power' are the first to lose sight of the true nature of helping others to heal, which is humbling and compassionate work. Once you begin to work with healing, you will find that simply being involved in an animal's recovery or restoration to health is such a deep privilege that all your own feelings, thoughts and worries are simply forgotten.'

HEALING YOUR PET

You can give healing energy therapy to your own pets at home as a way to help them recover from sickness, or to maintain their health. Of course, if your pet suffers a major injury, infection or other serious condition, you should seek proper veterinary attention. But the beauty of healing is that you can give it to your pet at any time, even on the way to the vet, to help ease shock and pain and boost the body's natural healing processes. You don't need to worry that you have no medical knowledge, because giving healing can benefit your pet whatever his condition – and you can never do any harm, because the body draws energy only as it needs it. Therefore, it is always worth giving a healing treatment, because you never know what kind of benefits might result. Even if all you do is make your pet feel more comfortable and relaxed, that in itself is a positive benefit.

Working with energy is a very simple process. Ultimately, you will develop your own style of giving energy therapy simply through practice. Each animal is an individual and each treatment will vary according to that individual's needs at the time. However, you have to start somewhere. All you need to do is remain aware of the feedback from the animal you're working on and trust your feelings and instinct to guide you. With small animals, you don't need to worry too much about were you place your hands because, although it helps to give as direct a 'hit' of energy as possible to the area requiring treatment, the body will draw energy to wherever it is needed. Besides this, when you're working on a little animal like a rabbit, say, there isn't much room to move your hands around.

PRACTICALITIES OF TREATING

Before you begin to work, it is as well to bear in mind a few practicalities about the conditions under which you give healing. Always remember that your pet should decide his treatment programme, not you, and that you need his 'permission' to treat him. He has to want to be healed.

Opposite. Scanning the body of the animal to identify weaknesses or blockages in its system. Rest your hands a few inches above the surface of the skin, drawing them down the body towards the legs and the tail.

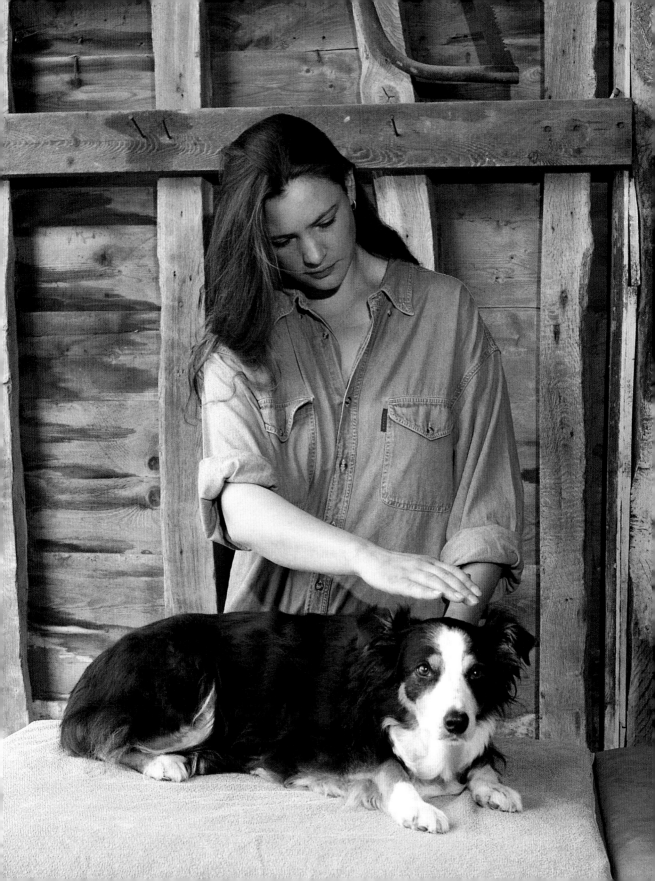

◆ Before you start, try to ensure that conditions are as comfortable as possible for you and your animal. For small pets such as cats, small dogs, rabbits; guinea pigs and other rodents, or for birds, you can simply lay a blanket or cloth over your lap or on a working surface at a suitable height, such as a table, and work on the animal in this way. Some subjects may prefer to be treated on the floor. If a cat or a dog is really sick it's easier to work on them wherever they sleep, and for animals like rabbits or rodents that are afraid of being handled, you can just place your hands around them in their cage or hutch. For reptiles, fish and animals, who live in regulated environments all you can do is adjust your treatment practice to suit the animal – so for a fish, you will need to place your hands gently around its body in the water.

◆ Try to ensure that other pets who can cause a distraction are kept away, but at the same time don't distress the animal you are working on by separating him from his companions. In an ordinary, domestic situation, you can simply treat your family dog or cat as he lies quietly on the floor or sofa without disrupting the normal routine too much.

◆ Treatments given indoors should go on as uninterrupted as possible. Make sure you can be free of disturbances such as the telephone ringing and away from noise from the television or radio. Household members should be asked to remain still and quiet, or to leave the room while you work, as their movement risks disturbing the animal you are working on.

◆ Make sure that food is not on the agenda – i.e. that no one is cooking, eating or preparing food for themselves or for animals. This kind of distraction is unfair if you're working on an animal that needs to relax during treatment.

◆ Large animals, such as farm animals and horses, should, whenever possible, be treated in the comfort of their own stall or stable. It is advisable to have a halter of some kind on the animal, as a safety precaution. You may need to move the animal to prevent it from treading on your feet, searching your pockets for food, nuzzling you or biting. It can also help initially to give some security where animals are nervous of being touched, until they have learned to trust you. Sometimes it can be helpful if there is someone to hold or move the animal, should it prove necessary.

◆ So that you can concentrate, it is as well to choose a time of day when the animal won't be waiting for a feed, exercise or some other kind of event that is part of its daily routine. You should be able to work with as little distraction as possible.

◆ The area you work in should be relatively clean and have adequate bedding for the animal to lie on during or after treatment, should it become drowsy. It should be fairly well sheltered from the weather. If necessary, use fly repellent to prevent the distraction of insects buzzing around and irritating both you and the animal.

◆ Your choice of clothing should be comfortable enough to work in for anything up to ninety minutes. In winter, you need plenty of layers. Coats made of fabric that crackles or rustles can startle the animal you're working on unless it's used to it; and your footwear should be comfortable enough to stand in for the duration of the treatment. You may need to take off your watch, if you find that working with energy affects it.

◆ You can never do harm by giving healing energy treatments. However, in the case of injuries such as pulled muscles or tendons, broken bones or open wounds, you should wait until the injury has been correctly set, bandaged or stitched by your vet before giving a full treatment. You should always place your hands to the sides of any injury to encourage correct natural cellular formation.

◆ If you feel there could be some risk to yourself in handling any animal, you could offer the healing from a safe distance. Signs of aggression in your subject may mean that the animal does not want to be treated.

ASSESSING ENERGY

Some people like to use tools such as pendulums to help them dowse the body. When you work with energy, this is quite unnecessary. In fact, the main purpose served by a pendulum is simply to amplify what the person using it, at some level, already knows or is aware of. With healing, it makes sense to remain uncluttered by props and simply to scan the body with your hands as a way of assessing where you need to place your hands and work.

To scan the body, rest your hands a few inches above the surface of the skin, as explained in Chapter 2, (see picture on page 35). It is best to start at one end, ideally at the head. Smoothly and steadily draw your hands down the body, moving towards the lower end of the body, the tail and feet. All the time, remain aware of any change of feeling in your hands as the body begins to pull energy more strongly in one area than another, or where the feeling changes. At first, you will simply find yourself naturally coming to rest over places where the body pulls energy strongly, or stopping where an area feels strange to you.

Scanning in this way can lead or alert you to areas that need treatment. It is essential always to keep an open mind when assessing your pet's energy in this way and not to be clouded by what you may have been told about a particular problem. Scanning the energy of the body can bring up new areas that need treatment which may hitherto have gone unnoticed through conventional methods of assessment or diagnosis. This is also why it is essential to begin to treat without bringing your own conditions or agenda to the treatment. You may find that you start working to treat a back problem only to find that the area that needs most work is the mouth, or the feet, for example. Conditions that first appear clear-cut can have causes related to quite another area of the body, so keep an open mind as you begin to work.

Scientists interested in energy exchange now believe that the process of energetic communication with another body, and the impressions and information received during treatment, takes place at a much deeper level of human awareness than we would usually make use of. You may, in fact, find yourself almost 'drifting off' as you scan or treat, as your level of awareness shifts to connect with the energetic transaction that is taking place. It's not uncommon to receive impressions about the condition you are working on, how it might have been caused or what can be done to help resolve it. This is simply the brain's way of making sense of the energetic information it receives – but more of this in Chapter 7.

You can begin to treat as you scan, or you can scan first and make a mental note of areas that feel different, before commencing treatment. A healthy body will simply feel warm under your hands and there will be nothing to alert you to any particular change in the feeling of energy being gently drawn into the body through your hands. Where areas feel particularly hot, this is usually the feeling of a greatly increased pull of energy coming through your hands, in other words

When treating a small and timid animal, like a rabbit, you can do it in its hutch or on your lap, if he'll let you, like the co-operative individual on the right. Hold your hands a little distance from the fur so that the animal does not overheat.

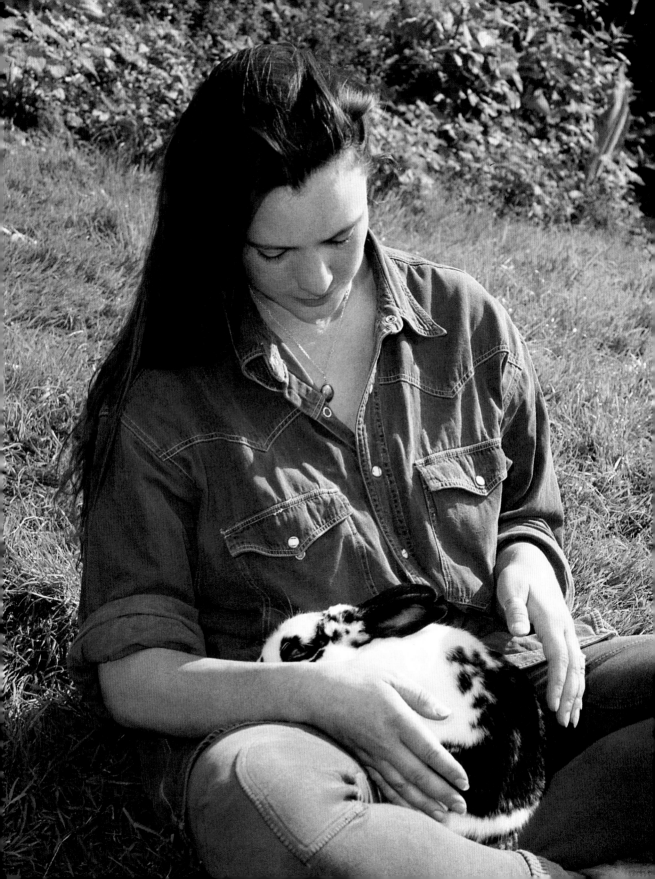

this is an area which needs treatment. Such areas may also feel thin or weak under your hand, which is usually an area either recovering from or approaching energy deficit. Where there are current or recent injuries, the area above the body might feel somehow tense, thick or congested. Areas of chronic pain or very old injuries which have never healed properly often feel cold and are completely blocked to any fresh input of energy. Blockages like these can take some time to shift. Each of these areas should be treated until the energy feels uniformly warm and smooth under your hand.

Because animals use their bodies to communicate with us, you should also remain aware of the reactions of the animal you are working on as you scan its energy. Animals know immediately what you're doing and so will react as they need to, in order to make sure they get the treatment they want. They will often move around to place the part of their body that most needs treating directly under your hand. They will shuffle, twitch, repeatedly look round at an area of their own body and even use their feet or head to push your hand to where they do, or don't want treatment. When you reach the place that is most in need of healing energy, most animals will relax and become very still and sleepy under your hand. If they really don't want to know, they'll either nip you or simply walk away!

The animal's natural response to treatment should not be suppressed – in other words, don't restrain it (unless it is simply nervous or fearful at first), or try to force treatment upon it. These reactions are actually of benefit to you, because they are genuine responses to the feeling of energy flowing into the body. For example, a dog that repeatedly touches his hip as you scan may pull in a vast amount of energy to his hip during treatment, indicating that the area is in need of healing. It is therefore as well to give animals as much scope as possible for movement as you scan, provided of course that you aren't going to be bitten or scratched! It can take some patience to scan or treat dogs that like to mouth, mainly because they will insist on picking your hands up constantly. The same applies to any animal that rolls over, and to cats that like to pat your hands and fingers. It can be difficult at first to distinguish between an animal's play antics and one who is trying to direct you to a part of their body that needs healing. With patience, you will find that attempts at play will generally cease after a while if you do not respond, whilst genuine efforts to direct you to part of the body that hurts will become stronger and more insistent.

By not restraining the animal, you always ensure that the treatment is actually wanted. Nobody has the right to force a treatment on an animal, or to say what treatment the animal should have other than the animal itself. So often I am asked to treat an animal because the owner is looking for a certain result – for their dog to calm down, their cat to get well, or their horse to do something it isn't necessarily happy to do. We have to remember that it's not up to us to decide the results we get, any more than it is the treatments an animal receives. People are often disappointed when their pet clearly is not interested in having healing – though this doesn't happen very often. Generally, animals will engineer a situation so that they get the treatment they need, whether by simply coming and making it obvious that they want your attention, or simply by being unwell. Animals who have science-defying conditions are often the ones who prompt their owners to seek alternative approaches like healing – and are very happy to receive their treatments. However, it is always as well to make sure and to mentally 'ask permission' before interfering with another body!

GIVING A TREATMENT

To begin treatment, you can simply place your hand anywhere on the body and project energy in. With animals that are so small your hands effectively cannot move into too many different positions, you can simply place your hands wherever it is most comfortable for you and your pet, and give them a treatment this way. However, for animals the size of a large rabbit or cat, a dog, or other larger creatures, it can help to have a set of hand positions to work through. In this way, you can address and treat all the areas you noted as you scanned the body. The hand positions given on page 43 address the main energy centres or chakras of the body, as well as the primary meridians or energy channels.

Bear in mind that you may need to adjust the height of your hand from the body as you work. Often a good way to begin working is to place the hands directly on the body, but the warmth of the energy can overheat some animals, so you may need to work a few inches away. Cats, in particular, are extremely sensitive to healing energy and some can find direct contact overwhelming. You will learn to experiment and adjust your working positions accordingly.

The easiest way to begin treatment is to make a connection and establish energy flow firstly in the area of the shoulder. This is usually a fairly 'safe' area to begin. Many animals will respond to the first feeling of energy treatment by

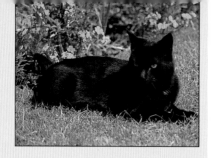

Fleur's flying lesson

Fleur is a two-year-old, green-eyed, black cat who was re-homed from an animal rescue centre. Fleur was quite thin when she moved to her new home, but had a lovely, affectionate nature and soon thrived.

One day her new owners came back to find her sprawled on the lawn in front of the house, clearly shocked and dazed, with the lady from next-door standing over her. The neighbour explained that, as she walked past, she saw Fleur looking out of an upstairs window, head and front paws on the outside, looking very comical. The neighbour had stopped to talk to Fleur and as she did so, Fleur – perhaps attracted by the sound of cans in the lady's shopping bag – scrambled up onto the frame of the open window and launched herself at the neighbour. Fleur landed heavily on the ground on her side and was taking rough, shallow breaths.

Her owner immediately rang the vet, as well as her daughter, who is a healing energy therapist. The daughter worked on Fleur in the car, all the way to the vet. Luckily, Fleur hadn't broken anything, but she was lying motionless on the vet's table – roughly forty minutes after her fall, still receiving healing treatment – when she suddenly struck out and scratched the vet with a loud 'miaow', sat up, and began grooming herself. Everyone was stunned at her quick recovery, given the shock she had experienced such a short time before. Fleur had treatments for the next few days, and was soon up to her old tricks.

relaxing, becoming quiet and still, or gently dozing. However, this is not always the case and some animals won't relax too deeply until they have learned exactly what you are doing and how it feels. Some very active animals simply never relax. Physically, you might notice that the respiration rate decreases and that gut sounds increase. Dogs in particular tend to mumble and mouth a little, as they would when dropping off to sleep. Of course, the cat's favoured response is to purr, but some will relax so deeply that even purring seems an effort.

At this stage, simply remain calm and quiet and be patient, as your pet may well fidget a little before he relaxes. Generally you should keep your hands as still as possible, but if it helps the animal to relax you can make stroking motions, at the same time maintaining the flow of energy to the animal's body. Once you have made your connection and the energy is flowing freely, you can work through the following series of hand positions (though you may simply prefer to treat the areas that you noticed as you scanned the body prior to treatment). It is most important, however, that you simply remain aware of your pet's responses and where he is guiding you to place your hands, where the pull of energy is increased or decreased, or where your pet responds particularly strongly. You can treat injuries or particular problem areas simply by placing your hands gently either side of the area, on or slightly above the body.

ROUTINE HAND POSITIONS (See opposite and page 47.)

There is no set time for which you should stay in each position – simply wait for a few minutes until the flow of energy subsides and you feel that you have done enough. I always encourage students to work slowly and steadily, without rushing. Where you are working on an area of particular energy deficit or a blocked, cold spot, this can take some time. Blockages in particular require patience as you wait until the area begins to pull energy in, and then finally 'tops-up' and the flow gently subsides again. If you work with your hands on the body, it is advisable to keep one hand in contact with the skin at all times so that you don't disrupt the flow, or surprise your subject! Remember too, to visualize the animal you are working on as healthy, whole and well, which will add positive strength to the treatment you give. I find it helps to 'see' the animal playing or enjoying some activity that he normally loves when he's healthy. Once you have made contact with the shoulder and treatment is underway, you can either work up the neck to the head, or down the body. With domestic pets, I

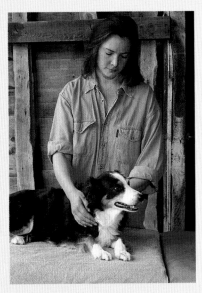

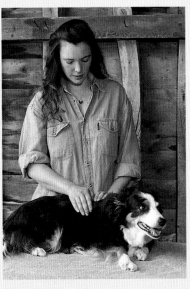

1 If your pet is happy for you to start treatment at the head, place one hand above it and one under his neck.

2 Move down to the shoulders or, alternatively start here if your pet finds it more comfortable. Place one hand on each shoulder.

3 Now start to work down towards the centre of the body.

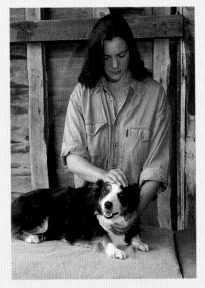

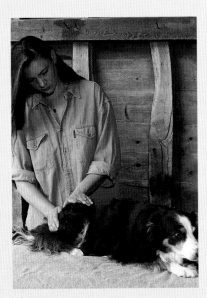

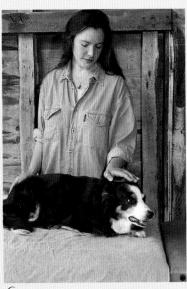

4 Keep your hands in the same position for a few minutes.

5 Work your way down towards the hips and the tail of the dog.

6 End the session of healing energy therapy with one hand at the base of the tail and one on the head of the animal.

generally work down the body towards the tail first, and finish by treating the head and neck. If you do start at the head, as I did with Pip on page 43, you are aiming to treat the energy centres of the head and throat first. Then, you can gradually work back down the body, stopping to work on the shoulders and heart area, solar plexus (below the ribcage), the centre of the body or navel area, the hips and loins, and the base of the tail. If your pet is lying down, he can be treated just as effectively – the energy will be drawn to the area of the body where your pet needs it most. You should avoid moving or turning the animal over during treatment as it is very disruptive. If the animal is sitting, like my dog Pip shown on the previous page, you can work with one hand on either side of the body. You can treat the legs without too much trouble as you move down the body. For cats and other small animals you may need to work 'hands-off' as they are very sensitive to energy and might feel rather hot.

With large animals like ponies, horses, and farm animals I tend to treat the head first, as this can help to relax and calm the animal (see page 47). Bear in mind that you will need to treat both sides of a large animal; in other words you will need to walk right round his body and finish back at the spot where you started. Start treatment at the shoulder, and work on one side of the body at a time. After the shoulder, you can work either on the throat and head, or down the body. Working downwards, you can rest at the heart, centre of the back and solar plexus or ribcage area, the navel region, the loins or hips, and base of the tail. Work down the legs on this side of the body, then go round and work up from the tail to the shoulder on the other side, and treat the legs on that side of the body. If you are finishing at the head, work on the neck and throat and then up to the jaw and forehead area before you finish. You will need to work down the legs, too, which is best done afterwards to minimize disruption to the flow of energy. Working through these positions ensures that you are treating the major energy systems. You will be working along the 'governing vessel', which is the major meridian along the top-line of the body, along the 'conception vessel', or major stomach meridian located along the underside of the body, as well as the locations of the seven main chakras or energy centres.

I recommend that you finish treatment at the 'top', in other words, at the head. By working down and up the body again, this helps to ensure that any areas of energy deficit are now healed. Remember to scan the body again as you finish treating, to ensure that there are no areas that feel uneven or still need treatment. A treatment on an animal that needs it can take up to ninety minutes. Small animals and those who are not too poorly, or can only cope with a little treatment at a time, may only need ten minutes work. Working with energy, however, is all about reading the body you are working on and following your instinct, so forget timing, treat your pet and be guided by his reactions.

HOW WILL YOUR PET RESPOND?

Many animals find that a treatment with healing energy therapy is so relaxing, that they simply fall asleep (such as my horse on page 46). With large animals you need to be certain that they can lay down in safety if they need to. If they do lie down, you can continue to work so long as you are careful not to put yourself in a position where you could be trodden on should the animal be startled into getting up suddenly.

The healing process can involve all kinds of releases during treatment. With people, the release is generally verbal as well as physical, as they talk about their feelings and thoughts during treatment. With the majority of animals, however, the releases during and after treatment are physical and include yawning, stretching, rolling, shaking, grumbling and afterwards, urinating.

Sometimes as you work on your pet he might revert to infantile behaviour such as making sucking motions with his mouth, or gentle paddling with the feet. Cats, particularly, do this as they become accustomed to treatment. This is indicative of an animal in a deeply relaxed state, experiencing treatment with energy as the same comforting feeling he would have received through close contact with his mother, very early in life.

It is advisable to monitor the animal you have treated for, say, ten minutes after you have finished working. Make sure that they have access to a drink and are warm and comfortable enough to go and find somewhere to lie down if they feel sleepy. Some very active dogs will respond in the opposite way, by going for a good romp accompanied by lots of loud barking!

TREATMENT SUMMARY

◆ Use the hand positions if you feel comfortable doing so. If not, let the animal you are working on and your intuition guide you. Some of the most powerful treatments are given by following the animal's reactions and you can easily spend half an hour working on, say, just the head, or the navel area.

> *'Many animals find that a treatment with healing energy therapy is so relaxing, that they simply fall asleep.'*

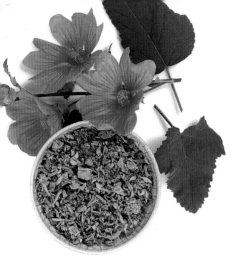

Marshmallow (*Althaea officinalis*). This plant is a great stand-by for coughs, colds and catarrh. It is available dried or can be gathered from the wild. Please note that the specimen shown is tree-marshmallow which makes an attractive garden shrub.

During an energy therapy treatment the subject often experiences total relaxation and may even fall asleep.

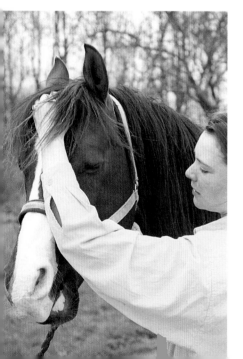

◆ In a first-aid situation, simply touch the animal in a part of the body that hasn't been hurt to give healing, and seek the correct medical attention. Giving energy to any part of the body will help to calm and soothe, as well as kick-starting the healing process.

◆ Injuries such as pulled muscles and tendons, burns, sores, broken bones and wounds should always be treated from the sides. If the animal you are working on is in pain or is extremely sensitive to touch, you can give a treatment by working with your hands a few inches off the body. This also applies to animals that might find the warmth generated by your hands a little too much to cope with.

◆ You can treat your pet as often as you feel he would like you to do so. For diseases, injuries or other conditions that you are working to help heal, it is advisable to treat daily from the outset, and if possible, twice a day, in the morning and evening. Remember that if your pet doesn't need or want a treatment, he'll soon let you know. There is no harm in offering energy, so don't be afraid to do it.

◆ You can give healing energy treatments alongside any other kind of treatment, therapy or medication, conventional or otherwise. It will simply serve to enhance the effect of any other treatment being given. Post-operative recovery can be greatly aided by giving regular energy treatments.

◆ Remember that legally, you cannot diagnose, and you should not work on animals belonging to other people without insurance. The person who cares for the animal should be aware that it is his or her responsibility to inform the animal's veterinary surgeon about any treatment given to the animal.

EVERYDAY ENERGY

Although the guidelines given here are for a formal treatment, if ever your pet is unwell, one of the great pleasures of working with energy is that you can simply incorporate it as part of your everyday life, every time you touch your pet. Most people who work with energy will simply treat their own animals in the evening as they sit and enjoy each other's company, perhaps by stroking a cat on your lap, whilst grooming, during handling, or just giving the dog a cuddle. I find that my

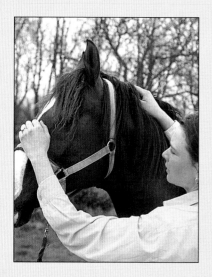

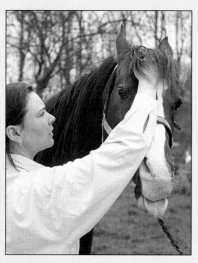

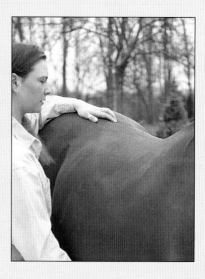

1 Begin working from the head, provided your horse is not head-shy. Keep a hand on his neck, this will help calm him.

2 Horses often yawn, lick or chew as they relax. Spend some time with your hand at his poll (top of the head).

3 Work gradually back along the body. You'll need to treat both sides of the body in turn.

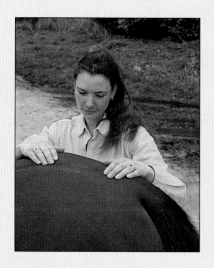

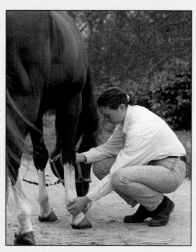

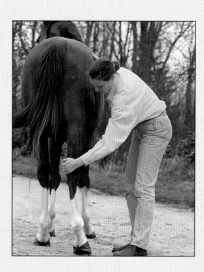

4 Continue, giving the spine special attention, and finish work on the body of the horse as you reach his hindquarters.

5 After working on the body, treat the front legs if necessary.

6 Finally, repeat the operation for the back legs.

hands are 'on', in other words I'm sending out healing energy, almost constantly, so when my dogs or horses feel they need some healing, they simply come and get it. Last thing at night, when we are all relaxing, I tend to 'plug' one hand in to each dog and simply doze off – it's a great way of ensuring a peaceful night's sleep for all of us. Remember that your pet will always benefit from a healing energy treatment – so don't limit treatments to times of sickness or convalescence. You can help maintain your pet's health and wellbeing by giving treatments as part of his daily routine. You can also use treatments to help clear a negative behavioural condition, for example to relax and calm your pet if he is scared of a particular situation.

While you are working on your animal, remember that you, too, are receiving some energy as it passes through you. This can be most beneficial for pet owners who are stressed or worried, for example, by their animal's illness, or made nervous by a behavioural problem.

IMPORTANT: The information given here is not intended as a substitute for veterinary advice or treatment. It is illegal for anyone other than a veterinary surgeon to diagnose, prescribe for or treat an animal. By law, the veterinary surgeon that normally treats an animal should be informed about any kind of complementary therapy that you intend to give your pet. Anyone giving therapy to an animal belonging to someone else should always make sure that they are adequately insured.

BEYOND THE HEALING TOUCH

HEALTH FOR LIFE

A therapy can only be of benefit if you make use of it. This might at first appear to be an obvious statement, but it is surprising how many people learn to use energy to heal and then only use it reactively – in other words, once a problem has occurred. One of the greatest advantages of working with energy to encourage natural healing is that you can give a treatment at any time of the day or night and as frequently or as rarely as you wish. One of the main values of energy therapy is that it can be used to bring the body back into balance and recharge existing energy levels. Therefore, it's not worth waiting until something has gone wrong in order to start giving treatment. Prevention, as always, is better than cure, and treatment can and should be given regularly and routinely to maintain your pet's health.

Domestic pets such as dogs and some cats, tend to lead quite active lives, as do their owners. Long walks, lots of healthy play for dogs and for cats, natural ranging behaviour and socializing with other animals, can result in wear and tear on the body. The fit, healthy body, with the advantage of youth, can cope perfectly well with life's daily stresses and strains. However, the cumulative effects of minor stresses over time can lay the body low and render it more open to sickness and other physical problems. Many injuries such as pulled muscles, ligaments and tendons are not just simply freak one-offs, but happen as a result of continued pressure on that part of the body, leaving it weaker and more prone to giving way under duress.

Viruses and infections can usually be fought off by an immune system that is functioning at optimum strength, but a weakened immune system is far more vulnerable to attack from the outside. It is vital, therefore, to maintain the body in optimum condition through good nutrition, a suitable environment and correct exercise levels. Don't make the mistake, though, of assuming that super-

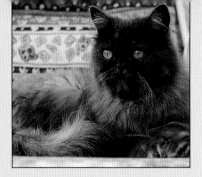

Tail tales

Sophie is an eleven-year-old Persian cat with a long, silky coat. She went missing for two days and her owners found her lying under the hedge, near the house . She had clearly been hit by a car and had struggled to get back to the house. After a visit to the vets, where she was cleaned and patched up, it seemed that, aside from the shock, cuts and bruises, the main injury was to her tail, which was severely out of line in several places. As a result, she couldn't find her balance and was having difficulty moving around normally. The vet said that, if Sophie didn't improve, the best option would be to remove her tail. However, he thought that she might learn to move normally if she could adapt to her new tail-shape. In time, the offending tail might even straighten up.

The difficulty was that Sophie seemed quite depressed and almost fearful of moving around. She just sat in her basket looking dejected. She had a half-hour healing treatment every other day for a week. After the second treatment, she started to be more confident and energetic, and began moving around a little more. By the second week, she was learning to cope, and, as the vet had hoped, the shape of the tail began to improve. Her owner learned to use healing energy treatment in order to go on helping the cat. Sophie is now just as agile as any other cat and the slight kink in her tail is the only reminder of her misadventure!

fit is also super-healthy. Some dog owners take great pride in giving their canine companions marathon-length walks and maintaining a rock-hard physique, but a body under great pressure to maintain an excessive level of exercise can often be stressed and more vulnerable to disease. Dogs should be got fit steadily and in stages – as should their owners. Animals kept for breeding, or in close confines with lots of other animals, are also more susceptible to the natural transference of organisms between them – which can include viruses as well as parasites.

Pets who are not kept in a controlled environment, in other words who have contact with other animals and the freedom to roam outside, are vulnerable to all kinds of other factors that can put pressure on the healthy body. These might vary from scavenging in unsavoury places, for example, to fighting for territory with a neighbouring animal, and avoiding predators or heavy traffic, particularly in busy cities. Similarly, physical and mental stresses are placed on animals whose natural ranging behaviour is curbed through living in a restricted area – for example, in a flat. All of the stresses that your pet encounters can clearly have an effect on the body, even if this just means one very sleepy pet at the end of the day! The ability to top up energy levels and rebalance the body on a daily basis provides a great way to maintain health and wellbeing and to deal with minor issues as they occur, so preventing the escalation into a more serious physical condition. It's also worth bearing in mind that if your pet suffers from a recurring condition that isn't

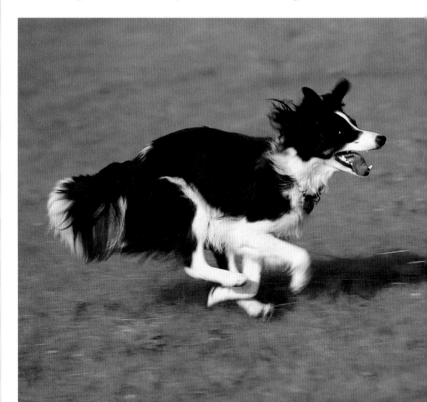

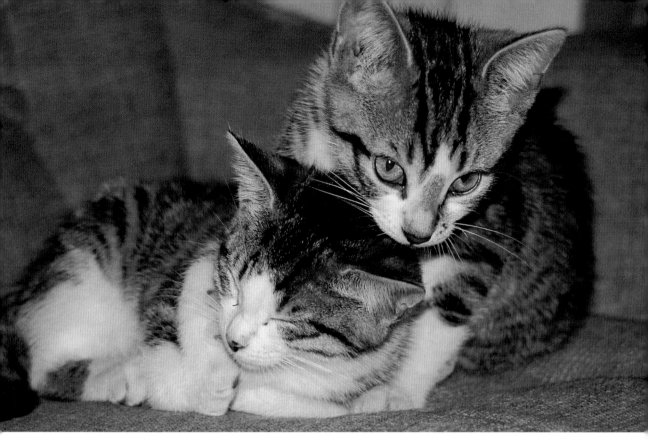

usually treated until it has manifested, you should be working to address the factors causing the imbalance and so prevent the condition from occurring at all. In this way you can work to help your pet maintain optimum health on a long-term basis, which is what healing, in its truest and most holistic sense, is all about.

WHAT CONDITIONS CAN YOU TREAT?

Treatments with energy are incredibly potent, yet are non-invasive and work naturally with the body. Because of this there are probably few conditions that cannot be treated or, at least benefit from healing energy. My own experience of healing animals includes treatment of everything from wounds, fractures and broken bones; pulled or strained muscles, ligaments and tendons; digestive problems; skin disorders; joint and locomotive conditions (including degenerative disorders such as arthritis); hormone imbalances; infections and viruses such as kennel cough; asthma, bronchitis, allergies of all kinds; tumours; spinal curvature; to post-operative care and convalescence, and even just fatigue. I find that problems to do with the skeleton respond particularly well to healing. I have worked on countless cases of broken bones, including cat's broken tails,

Above. Touch and physical contact forms a vital part of a kitten's, or indeed any animal's growing up. Kittens lie down curled up against each other, a position which gives them comfort and a sense of security, even after they've been separated from their mother. This is one of the reasons why animals respond so well to energy therapy, with its emphasis on gentle touch.

Opposite. Working dogs, such as this border collie, need a tremendous amount of exercise and space around them or they will start behaving in a way which may cause their owners problems: rounding up the children, for instance, chasing other animals, or running into city traffic.

small breaks in the bones of dogs' feet, and chips and fractures in horses' legs that have recovered in a fraction of the time the vets expected them to. I recently worked on a dog with two fractured ribs who seemed to make a truly miraculous recovery – within a week of his accident he was back to his normal self and clearly pain-free. Lame cats, often suffering from muscular and ligament pain, possibly due to landing heavily or perhaps falling from a height – a very frequent cause of injury among cats living in tall buildings in cities – have arrived at my house hopping on three legs, and been sound the next day.

HELPING TO HEAL THE PHYSICAL

Pet owners tend to resort to alternative or complementary approaches, particularly to calling in a healer, when they feel they have exhausted every other possibility available to them. They believe that their animal is beyond help, but are nevertheless determined to 'give anything a go'. All kinds of physical conditions are called 'incurable'. For example, Toby, a thirteen-year-old Jack Russell terrier belonging to one of my clients, had suffered from both joint and muscular problems for many years. His vet had examined him time and time again, but there was nothing he could do to make life any easier for Toby. The little dog had recurring difficulty with one of his hips and often carried one hind leg off the ground for long periods of time, just hopping along. The day he came for healing, he was depressed and obviously in discomfort. He had a ninety-minute long treatment and fell asleep on my lap as I worked on him. Afterwards, he didn't want to go home. His energy levels improved dramatically the day after treatment and he was walking normally again on all four legs within a few days. He has a herbal mixture daily in his food to help maintain his ease of movement as part of his long-term healthcare.

Toby's story goes to show that there is more than one way to approach everything in the world, and sometimes it simply takes time to find the one that will work for you. Exhausting the possibilities available through one system is unlikely to mean that nobody, anywhere else, could help. This is one of the main reasons why I believe that healing energy therapy should be given unconditionally and with the intent of helping the animal to heal as is best for that individual. It is important that, no matter what label has been given to the condition you are treating, you simply offer energy and focus on bringing the body back into balance and wholeness.

It isn't easy to ignore labels like 'incurable' or 'terminal'. However, it can help to work on developing a little detachment from the problem in hand, in order to offer energy and give the body the opportunity to do with it as it will. This is also essential because of the inextricable link between the condition of the mind and body, so that what might first seem to be purely a physical condition may have quite other origins, which I will explain in more detail later. Aside from this, as I mentioned in Chapter 3, what first appears to be a problem with one part of the body can be related to or caused by something happening elsewhere. Other conditions may have gone undiagnosed due to slight, but obscure imbalances or physical disruptions that remained undetected.

Sometimes, one problem can go untreated for some length of time because the therapeutic focus is on another, where the two may in fact be closely related. For example, problems in the back and limbs are often connected – discomfort can easily be caused in the back muscles due to an injury in the leg affecting posture and movement. This is particularly true where animals have suffered a fall, and the back is treated because this is where the immediate and obvious effect of the accident is. However, when the condition clears up only to reoccur at a later date, one has to look elsewhere for another physical cause.

This is so often the case with ponies and horses who suffer direct injuries to the back during a boisterous chase in the field, a fall on the road or during cross-country jumping. The pony or horse in question is often immediately lame and the back clearly traumatized; following manipulation and rest, the animal is returned to work. Such ponies and horses can then suffer recurrent back problems, sometimes accompanied by obscure and fairly minor lameness, which becomes progressively worse with each episode. The whole problem can be related to hind leg trauma, in the stifle, hock or even the fetlock. The joint in question appears to have suffered low-level trauma during the original accident, but not enough to detract from the focus on the injured back. That trauma tends to become aggravated though work, and the pain can cause the horse or pony to compensate by changing its movement, which tends to create muscular soreness in the back.

I have also seen this problem in dogs and cats; in particular, one cat who had been hit by a car but appeared to have made a full recovery at the time, but who later began to move as if her back was permanently half-arched. In obscure or confused cases, healing energy therapy can be given to the animal to encourage

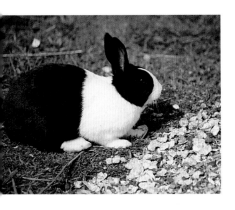

Below. The benefits of healing energy can be enjoyed by owner and pet as part of a grooming or a play session. Giving healing energy will soon become part of the daily routine for both of you and your pet may even be disappointed when touched by someone whose hands do not provide it.

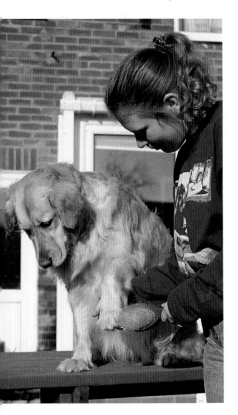

healing of the whole condition, whether other contributory factors have been recognized or not. I have worked on several cases where locomotive problems have been given up on because the root cause of the condition was elsewhere in the body but had simply not been identified. Toby, the little Jack Russell I mentioned earlier, had an area of blocked energy forward of his pelvis, which was clearly related to his lameness – it turned out that he had suffered a twisting fall some years before that had resulted in some lameness at the time, but nothing remarkable. In some animals, lameness can even come from pain in the head. I treated a little cat who had a growth in her mouth that couldn't be seen from outside – the pain caused her to carry her head very slightly to one side and she became more and more sore in her front leg. In circumstances such as these, a truly holistic way of treating has some advantage over the symptomatic approach. All of these situations and possibilities add weight to the principle of working to offer energy not just, for example, for the back problem, or for the lameness, but for the whole animal.

THE HOLISTIC NATURE OF BEING

It is all very well to consider the ways in which you can help to heal your animals' physical conditions. However, the point is that each and every condition that our bodies manifest is likely to have its roots in something that is going on mentally. Conversely, behavioural issues – those that are said to be 'all in the mind' – have frequently been caused by some kind of physical trauma. There are borderline conditions where the distinction between physical and mental becomes quite blurred. For example, in cats and dogs, fur-licking and excessive self-grooming can be the symptom of an allergy, an injury or even comfort behaviour related to nervous tension; the same is also true of horses with the equivalent equine habits of excessive scratching and rubbing, or even coat and skin-biting. The same principle applies to some digestive disorders. It is essential, therefore, to consider the cyclic inter-relationship of mind and body as you work with energy to encourage healing.

Physical conditions that may have a mental factor involved include those where the animal has succumbed to sickness due to the immune system being suppressed, through stress. This might, for example, take into account dogs and cats that succumb to kennel cough and other infections upon leaving animal shelters. The stress of being abandoned or ill-treated, housed in a communal shelter or kennel for some time, and then re-homed can all lower the body's natural ability to fight off infection. It may also, as I mentioned earlier, take into account those animals that are over-exercised, such as some working dogs, which may have insufficient time for rest or play. It can also include animals on the show circuit, who are often kept cosseted with constant grooming, yet with little natural exercise, and lots of stressful travel to shows.

Other physical conditions where mental factors have been brought into play include animals that repeatedly suffer from injuries due to falls, becoming trapped or through fighting. In such cases, by treating your pet with healing energy, you will be helping to heal the 'personality' behind the problems, as well as the result of the physical actions. For example, dogs who are easily excitable, always rushing everywhere and prone to sudden bursts of frenetic activity, are often the ones who suffer accidents through chase or fall injuries. We've all seen the young or adolescent dog who suddenly, with alarming regularity, takes off round the place at exuberantly high speed (what I call the 'wall of death' syndrome!), only to fall panting to the floor within a few minutes. Often this kind of frenzied excitement results in a poorly pup with a knock on the head from having run into something, or a twisted ligament through having turned too sharply. Some cats will behave in a similar way if in company with other youngsters, flying up and down anything vertical and occasionally falling off it in the process. Whilst this kind of behaviour is a sign of a healthy, energetic animal, the injuries that can result are rarely to the animal's benefit. In cases like these it can help to give the animal in question regular treatments to help to maintain a calm, relaxed outlook and to balance the sudden surges of energy that contribute to this behaviour.

Behavioural problems caused by physical factors are often the result of previous unhappy experiences, simply because of the way that the brain learns through stimulus-response conditioning. For example, some animals might exhibit nervous, aggressive or anxious behaviour due to what I call a 'memory-scar'. A simple example of this might be the cat who keeps out of the kitchen because he once burned his feet by walking on the still-hot oven. He experienced pain in that situation and the trauma of that memory has been stored in the brain, affecting his future behaviour. This is fine unless he has to pass through the kitchen to leave or enter the house! Other examples might include animals with stress-related behaviours of some kind that are related to

Lester, the rescued rabbit

Twelve-year-old Fiona acquired her rabbit, Lester, from an animal shelter, where he had been taken by a family whose children had lost interest in him. Lester was very thin indeed, his nails had been allowed to get far too long, he had skin problems and his coat was badly matted. The shelter had asked the vet to cut his nails and attend to his skin, but Fiona now had to groom him regularly to get his coat back into condition, and ensure that he ate and drank properly.

Although Lester was soon eating well, Fiona had real trouble handling him as he wasn't used to it. She got scratched every time she tried to touch him, and spent a long time chasing him round the hutch before she could catch and groom him. Fiona's dad got round the problem by making a special hutch in which the sides simply unclipped. Fiona could lift the front and sides out, one by one, making access easier, but leaving Lester inside his hutch.

Fiona's father was a therapist who worked with energy, giving healing to people as his full-time job. He and Fiona worked on Lester together. Fiona would offer some dandelion leaves to Lester while her dad unclipped three sides of the hutch; meantime, Lester felt safe and happy, munching on his leaves against one wall. Then, while Fiona gently worked on Lester's coat, her dad moved his hands around Lester's body to give him a treatment at the same time. This helped the rabbit to stay calm as well as to improve his health.

Gradually, they began moving Lester from the hutch to Fiona's lap for his grooming and treatment and after a while, Fiona was able to handle him and groom him. Lester's health and weight improved and his coat was soon smooth and glossy. He is is now tame enough to play in Fiona's bedroom as she does her homework.

previous experience; who are afraid of humans, of being left alone, of water, of travelling in the car, or of other animals. I have seen one dog who was happy with his owner until she bought a new overcoat, when he panicked – not at his owner, but at the coat, wherever it was left in the house. Horses, particularly, carry such 'memory-scars' with them for years, and their fears are often related to the pain caused by ill-fitting saddles, which can result in aggression towards anyone carrying a saddle. All of these behavioural patterns evolve through physical experience and learning.

Situations such as these can prove confusing if behavioural patterns or physical problems are considered in isolation, and can lead even some of the most effective orthodox approaches to draw a blank. However, where healing energy therapy is concerned, because of the whole-individual way in which it works, all of these issues can gain some real benefit. Sometimes this only becomes apparent as treatment progresses – the animal stops doing something it's always done, or just learns to relax. The traumas held in the mind, that in turn produce the behaviour that we might find difficult to live with, can be gently released as the animal learns to relax and gradually adopt new behaviours.

Healing for behavioural problems is of great benefit to animals who change hands once or more during their lives, especially if they have been through an animal shelter, and might come to you with all kinds of habits that you just don't understand. My experience includes treating dogs who destroy the house when their owners leave them alone; dogs who stray; cats who refuse to be handled at all, or that become 'aggressive' when handled; cats and dogs who panic when the vacuum cleaner is turned on, or when there are men or children around. I have worked on horses that are aggressive, or terrified of people; or that appeared impossible to train. I have worked on dogs, cats, horses (and even rabbits) that exhibit all kinds of behaviour related to individual fears and traumas. Again, the list of conditions associated with treatment is endless, but whatever the condition, you can give treatments regularly to help your pet to cope with whatever the situation is that he finds difficult.

HEALING BEHAVIOURAL PROBLEMS

One of the main reasons that animals respond so well to healing energy therapy is that it is completely non-invasive and involves nothing more complicated than the touch of your hand. Touch provides a universal form of essential communication between species, and because it forms the basis of much of the natural language of our animals, touch therapies feel safe, comforting and natural to them. Using energy through touch can therefore provide the key to facilitating the healing of behavioural problems in our pets. Where learning has led to a negative or traumatic memory related to a particular stimulus, animals (including ourselves) continue to repeat the same related behaviour in any situation that triggers that memory. Often the playing out of behaviour takes place in total absence of anything approaching the original stimulus.

Behavioural 'problems' are not, generally speaking, a problem for the animal concerned – but they can present difficulties for the humans who live with that animal – think of the cat with the sore paws, who is afraid of going into the kitchen! Behaviours that make life difficult, such as these, often respond to healing energy therapy simply because it can have such a deeply relaxing effect on the animal being treated. This has to be one of the gentlest ways to help any animal to learn – without force, without restraint, fear or domination.

A key way to use energy to help release behavioural problems is to relax and calm your pet, so that he can learn about new situations. This is extremely helpful if your pet is nervous, for example during potentially stressful situations, such as when going to the vet for inoculations, or when travelling in the car for the first time. Giving energy to your pet in situations that could easily become negative and fearful, can turn the experience into a simple, stress-free occasion. Knowing the value of learned behaviour, this is one way in which energy can actually be used as a training aid, particularly for young animals or those new to the household. By approaching each new situation in a calm and settled way, you will soon have a calm and settled pet.

Where old habits and memory scars are concerned, the first step in using healing energy to help to heal the memory and thus to retrain your pet is to become aware of the ways in which your pet communicates with you. The easiest way for us to understand our pets is through their body language. This forms a large part of their communication with each other, and provides a key for us in understanding what they are trying to tell us.

IS YOUR PET TELLING YOU SOMETHING?

Our animals are communicating with us constantly, whether we are aware of it or not. What they do or 'say' only tends to become glaringly obvious, however, when it creates a situation we find difficult to live with. Cats, particularly those who tend to remain somewhat separate or isolated from their human companions, can sometimes be more difficult to understand than dogs, which are more demonstrative and obvious about what's troubling them. One of the main reasons 'problem' cats can be difficult to relate to is because they're not home very much, and when they are, they're sleeping! Basically, as humans (and therefore a different species than our pets), we're suffering from a simple case of language barrier. It's a bit like the classic situation where we go abroad and shout, in our own language, at a native of the country we're visiting, desperate to make ourselves understood. How frustrating! We have all seen or been involved in situations like these, where we just can't explain what we mean (and end up with a salad instead of soup!). In situations like these even humans resort to body or sign language.

It's one thing to be involved in an interaction with another human being who is aware that we're trying to get our message across to them, to make ourselves understood. But our animals can get stuck by being ignored or at worst, told off,

We all love our dogs, but misunderstand their language. We see licking as a 'kiss' or a sign of particular affection, when in fact the dog may be merely asking for food.

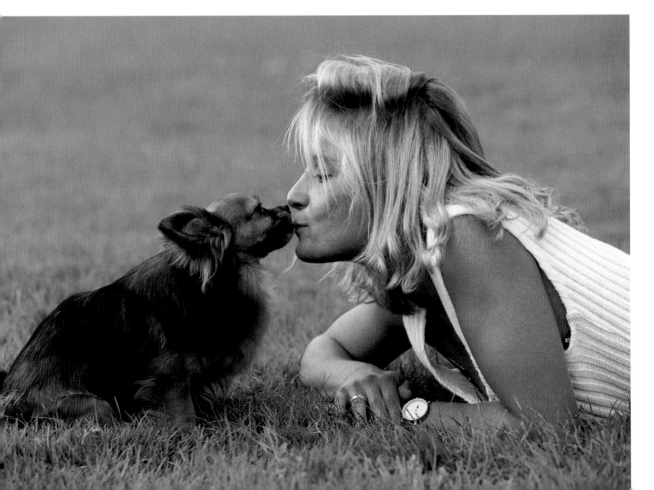

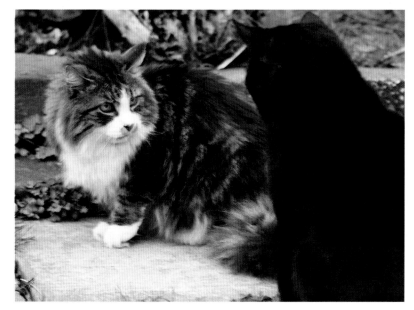

Two cats who do not know each other and meet in a garden, for instance, use body language to determine 'who is boss' and establish their respective territories.

as we misunderstand what it is they're trying to communicate to us. Imagine always ending up with a salad and never getting the soup! The problem, in fact, is not what the animal is doing – just that we don't know how to make sense of his behaviour. The favourite phrase that confused humans use, when all else fails, is that their pet has 'just started doing something'. They usually tag on, 'for no reason at all'. No reason at all? It's surprising how often we apply this phrase to animals but not to other people. Because, of course, we wouldn't start 'doing something' for no reason at all, now would we?

Animals, humans included, don't 'just do things', and especially not without reason. At some level, every action and reaction is carried out as a means to continue existing. The language barrier we're up against means that the behaviour our animals exhibit is sometimes difficult for us to understand – but the motivation for their behaviour is always there. Humans are fairly isolated in the intellectual maze that surrounds our motivation and reasoning. Other animals tend to operate on a much clearer level and as such, much of what we attribute to our animals is somewhere between a huge stretch of the imagination, and a projection of our own thoughts and feelings. Animal behaviour is directly related to motivation from the environment (and the 'environment' includes factors like you). In other words, if an animal is hungry or thirsty, his behaviour will be that of an animal searching for food or water. If he's tired, his behaviour will be that of an animal seeking a safe place to sleep.

If he's scared, he'll do whatever comes naturally to help him to protect himself – whether that means fighting or running away and hiding.

Let's go back to our example of the cat who stood on the oven and burned his paws. The first thing you're aware of is that, for 'no apparent reason', he suddenly refuses to go anywhere near the kitchen. The problem with this is that the cat-flap in the kitchen door is his only means of entry to, and exit from, the house. All you might be aware of is that he's suddenly hanging about in the house, near the kitchen, whining away – he doesn't want food, he doesn't want to be picked up, and he doesn't want to go out because he isn't going anywhere near the door. This kind of behaviour may go on for some time until you finally decide it's time for the cat to go out. Then you either pick him up and put him outside, or coax him outside with a toy or some food. The next time you're puzzled is when he's hanging around outside the door whining, and seems to want to come in, but won't. So, you pick him up and carry him in. Pretty soon, your cat will learn to associate his behaviour with you carrying him in or out of the door. It's a neat way to get where he wants to go, but not always practical.

For the cat, this situation is not so bad after all (as long as you pick him up on cue), because he's avoiding the stove – the place which hurt and scared him. For you, it's pretty frustrating when you don't understand why he's 'just started doing this', why you have to keep carrying him in and out and why, if you don't get him out in time, he ends up using part of the house as a lavatory! He will quite likely start trying to find other ways to get in or out of the house. This might involve scratching up against the windows, running out of the front door, or jumping out of an upstairs window. Plenty of these apparently illogical and mysterious behaviours can be tracked back to one bad fright and the need to find a way round the object of fear. Sometimes, it's hard to do the detective work yourself and someone from outside the family or household might have a more detached view of the situation.

Your cat's behaviour seems more and more irrational, and gets more and more difficult to live with. You're perplexed because you didn't see him jump up onto the stove to investigate the source of the lovely smells following the preparation of the evening meal. You didn't see him getting his paws burnt as he landed on a hot-plate too quickly to realize it was still hot, and his flight across the room in a state of shock and panic. If you're lucky, you may, as you're carrying him you notice that his paws look a bit scorched. Or, you may look at his feet because he's walking gingerly or licking them a lot. He might scratch you as you carry him past the stove, or he might even have left some paw-prints on it. Any of these clues would help you to put two and two together.

A brave cat, or one pushed, by necessity, to venture back into the kitchen might get as far as approaching the stove to find out whether it's on or not before he goes any closer, or he may even rush past the stove in a panic. Alternatively he might just find somewhere comfortable to wait around outside the house until he knows you're around to let him in. A less brave cat or one who has been badly frightened, needs to learn that actually the kitchen is quite safe. His feet need to heal, and he needs to learn, gently and positively, that he can not only go back into the kitchen but that he can also walk past the stove and let himself in and out of his cat-flap again. The only lesson he should positively retain from all this is not to jump on the stove! One interesting point to note about this example is that your cat is not still having his feet scorched – but he remembers how it felt. He is still reacting to the original stimulus by carrying the memory of the fear and pain.

It is surprising how far animals will go to avoid pain – be it physical or emotional (this latter applies to us, too). Often, the fear of pain is enough to trigger the learned behaviour. It's fascinating how humans carry such 'memory-scars' with them and continue to exhibit learned behaviours in the absence of the original stimuli – which can prove to be either a positive, useful learning experience, or a negative habit, depending upon the circumstances involved.

LETTING GO OF FEAR

When faced with our problem cat – who is now doing all kinds of strange things except coming and going in the usual manner, and driving you crazy into the bargain – energy therapy can help him to heal in a number of distinct ways. First, nobody may even know about his scorched paws. If you scan his body with your hands, you will become aware of the places which pull in more energy than others – in this case, his poor feet. This would give you a good idea as to where the physical problem is that needs to be healed. So, you can treat him to help his feet to heal.

Then, whether you know about the stove incident or not, you can work to heal his mind and encourage him to let go of his fear. This is simply done by giving him a relaxing treatment at the same time as asking him gradually to venture into the kitchen. On a mental level, energy therapy promotes confidence and calm by inducing a state of relaxation in the brain. You may need to place yourself a little way inside the kitchen and sit and stroke him on your lap whilst giving him some energy; you may need to play with him, or feed him, at the same time as giving energy to his body as you stroke and talk softly to him. Little by little, you can move steadily further towards the door and past the stove, so that he gradually learns to remain relaxed, calm and happy and to let go of his fear. As this process takes place, he no longer needs to keep trying to find ways around the kitchen and so he forgets his other maddening behaviour.

This is just one example of the ways in which you can use energy to help to heal your pet's issues and to help to teach him new behaviour. All of this happened to my own cat, Ben, and I was stumped for days until I carried him past the stove one evening as I was cooking dinner, only to have him launch himself across the room. This kind of situation particularly applies to horses who become 'spooky' about certain gateways, places on the yard, and so on. One of my young horses, Ace, suddenly began to panic at a particular gateway and refused to go past it without a ten-minute session of comforting and persuasion, which I had to repeat for several days. When I investigated the gateway, it turned out that the electric fence was touching it very slightly, and only in one corner, but enough to electrify the whole gate! Ace had clearly had a shock as he waited to come in one evening and was justifiably avoiding the source of his fright.

The main aim is to keep your pet relaxed and calm, to help him to let go of his fear. This method can also be applied in situations where fear is not the issue, in other words where you want to teach your pet to replace one kind of behaviour with another. The situations in which you can apply this kind of work are limitless. For example, if you have a dog who is terrified of the vacuum cleaner, you can begin giving him energy therapy before putting the vacuum cleaner on, and you will find that he gradually learns to remain calm and let go of his anxiety over the problem. This is the kind of issue that many animal trainers would tackle simply through de-sensitizing, which sometimes has to be repeated again at a later date if, through lack of exposure to the problem stimulus, the animal simply becomes sensitized again.

To summarize, where behavioural issues are concerned, energy therapy can be used as a stand-alone treatment to relax and calm nervous, anxious, tense or stressed animals. It can be used in a calming or relaxing way as a preventive measure, for example, when travelling with a young animal for the first time, and for dogs, during the training process. It can also be used as part of the handling process, where animals have remedial problems that need to be released and retrained. You can use energy to calm any animal in a tense situation. these are some examples where healing energy will help your pet to cope with difficult or stressful situations:

To maintain calm, and as a preventative measure:

- For nervous, anxious pets.
- Where tension causes difficulties with handling or training.
- For pets who lack confidence.
- At a traumatic time, such as injury, accident or giving birth.
- Before leaving your pet alone for the first time.
- After a house move.
- Before, during and after visiting the vet.
- When visitors come to the house.
- At a show or out shopping.
- When clipping and grooming.
- When travelling.
- For socializing with other animals.
- For new pets and during training.

Working and show dogs love outings and can get really excited at the prospect. Offer energy to help balance and settle nerves or tension.

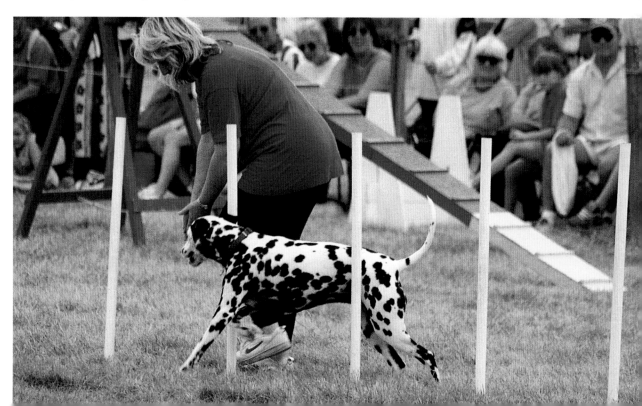

To help to release and clear problems such as:

◆ Biting.

◆ Aggression.

◆ Destructive behaviour and unwanted habits.

◆ Fear: of situations, places, other animals, objects, people, noises and so on.

MIRROR, MIRROR ...

The point to bear in mind when working with behavioural issues is that our pets frequently mirror our own behaviour. Thus it is common to see a pet that is stressed living with a stressed owner, and a pet that is very laid back living with a very laid-back owner. Some people buy or choose animals that reflect their own personalities, but some pets become that way through exposure to their owners. Other people project their own issues onto their animals. I have some clients who insist that their animals are stressed or sick when the animal is, in fact, fine while the owner is the one presenting problems.

Often it is difficult for people to believe or understand that the 'difficult' behaviour their pets display can be a reaction to what those humans are doing themselves. A little objectivity is most helpful in situations where you begin to suspect that in fact, your pet is reacting to you. I have even seen tense pet owners describe their pets as tense when in fact, the pets aren't tense at all – but the owner is! Most of the time, what people do with their own actions hasn't been carefully thought out in terms of how it might affect their pets – and this is perfectly normal. However, in situations where you're stuck with an animal that is doing something you don't understand and you're struggling to cope with it, it can be worth taking a look at how you are handling the situation.

Let's reconsider our scorched cat, for example. It is easy to imagine how, once the cat has started exhibiting all kinds of stressed behaviour (jumping out of upstairs windows, scratching at the door or window frames, using a corner of the carpet as his lavatory), the humans in that cat's life could respond by exhibiting some stressed behaviour, too! Telling the cat off, shouting at him, shutting him out or refusing to feed him unless he sits near the stove are all possible (but rather negative) reactions to what the cat is doing. His behaviour has resulted in a degree of stress to you. But negative reactions, like telling him off, are going to increase his stress levels too and then he's going to do something else – he might just decide not to come home, for example.

This is how animals and humans, struggling to overcome the language barrier, can suffer a breakdown in communication. Sometimes it's not even this complex – you might have just carelessly done something that triggered a change in your pet's routine, for example, and so he's reacting to that. This is what I call getting locked into the downward, stress-related spiral in the relationship between human and animal. If you're honest and take a good look at your own actions and reactions, you might find the way out. The beauty of working with energy is that you may well become more sensitive to and aware of situations such as these and learn to handle your pet differently, or learn to change whatever it is about your own behaviour that triggers you pet's stress reactions.

Because you are part of your animals' environment and he is part of yours, each of you has a significant influence upon how the other experiences the world. It can help to consider this as you work on healing behavioural problems because it is impossible to bring about a positive change without involving your own behaviour, too. Once the healing process begins, however, and a little light is shed on the situation, the turning point is reached where you can both begin to enjoy the journey back up the spiral towards a stress-free relationship. Generally this happens naturally – as your pet starts to heal, your stress levels are reduced, so your reactions to him are less stressed, so he feels happier, and so on. This is a great way to move forward together and learn from the situation – yet another example of how animals can teach us so much.

A COMPLETE APPROACH

Many of our animal's conditions that need healing can be treated purely with healing energy. However, it is unfair to expect healing with natural energy to act as a one-off, miraculous, instant cure-all. It has to be kept in context, and it can and should be used alongside other therapies, as and when appropriate. It may be advisable to work in conjunction with other experts, such as handlers, trainers and of course, the vet, to help your pet to heal. Sometimes, it can also be useful to consider other factors as part of the healing process. For example, it's no use blasting your pet with energy and expecting him to be well if you're not feeding him a balanced diet. Remember, though, that alternative medicines, including herbs, essential oils, homeopathy, Bach flower remedies and crystals, are symptom-oriented, just like synthetic remedies. It can therefore be helpful, whatever you choose, to incorporate energy therapy as part of a whole-system approach to healing for animals (and, of course, humans).

'Because you are part of your animals' environment and he is part of yours, each of you has a significant influence upon how the other experiences the world.'

ENERGY, FREQUENCIES AND VIBRATION

The effects of giving healing energy therapy to animals and people alike can be astounding. Because of this, there are practitioners who recommend that healing with energy be regarded as the only therapy you will ever need – a cure-all. This may well be true; however, it helps to maintain a balanced approach to working with energy and to treat it as part of your therapeutic tool-kit. Wise practitioners will recognize the benefits of all manners of therapy in helping the body to heal, as well as how different therapies can complement and boost each other's efficacy.

As we have seen, the use of energy as an integrated part of a total, holistic approach to healthcare is still practised in some parts of the world today and is based on age-old traditions. Most people are aware of the balancing principles of Yin and Yang, which can be expressed in many different ways, but are merely an expression of opposites in form. In eastern medicine, the body is balanced using the 'five elements' – water, metal, earth, fire and wood (or sometimes air). These elements may vary according to the tradition you follow. Ancient Greek healthcare was based upon the idea of 'humours' in much the same way, and other systems are concerned with balancing wet and dry (water and air) with cold and heat. Such principles have persisted through to recent and, in many cases, modern times as a means to keeping the mind and body in balance as a whole – through diet, exercise, and mental or spiritual exercises such as meditation.

Although the concept of the 'elements' is alien to most westerners, the basic idea is one of working to heal both mind and body continually in terms of nourishment, physical exercise, and mental wellbeing. If you translate this principle in its most basic terms to caring for your pets, you can't expect to maintain their health with energy therapy if their basic wellbeing, in terms of dietary requirements, exercise and so on, is not attended to.

Opposite. My Anglo-Arab mare, April Airs and her five-month-old foal, April Violet, which we are weaning naturally.

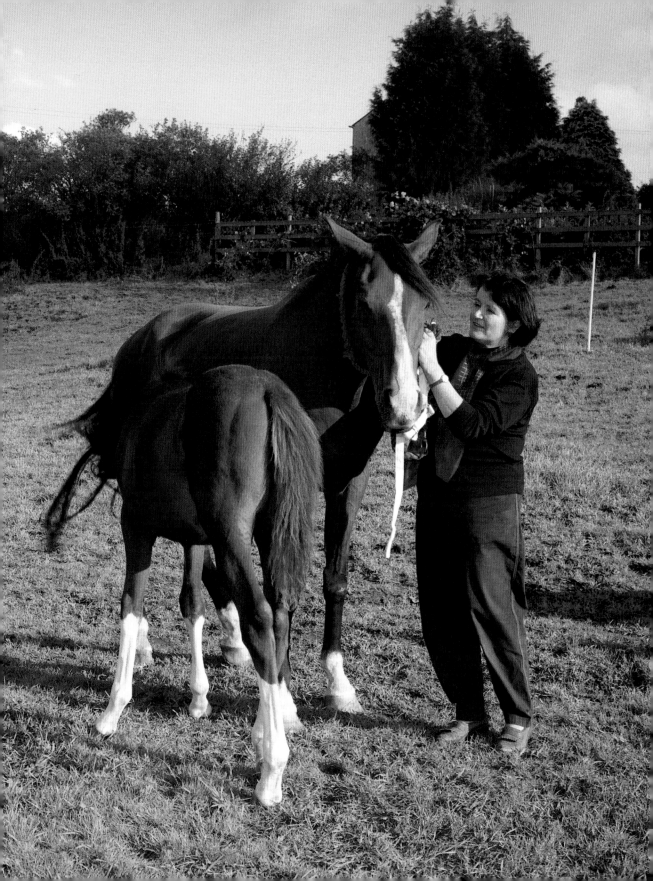

If you are treating your own pet, you will know him well enough to be aware of shifts, improvements, plateaus and changes as they take place. Often, the healing process happens through a series of improvements interspersed with plateaus or 'resting periods', where the body and mind assimilate the changes they are going through before moving forward again. Often the plateaus or phases of assimilation will signify the end of a useful period of one particular kind of treatment, and the beginning of another, as the body retains the benefit from each treatment and reaches a certain level of wellbeing. The assimilation phase between improvements can offer an opportunity to introduce new factors into the healing process. This is where the use of other forms of energy medicine, such as aromatherapy or homeopathy, can provide a key to the next phase of growth and healing, by raising the energy of the body to its next phase.

The timing between phases may be quite short, even just a few days, or it may be several weeks or months. It is therefore wise to introduce other forms of energy medicine to the healing process, one at a time, and to give each remedy plenty of time to work. Natural remedies can often need longer to take effect on the body than synthetic drugs, purely because they are working to boost the body's own healing mechanisms to overcome sickness, as opposed to sending in the troops for a quick fight before pulling out again! If you do use more than one remedy at once, you will have no idea what is producing the positive effect and you may even end up inadvertently counteracting the effects of one remedy with another.

So think carefully, make your choice and work with your chosen remedy until either some improvement is shown, or it is clear that your pet is gaining no benefit from what you are using. If you are in any doubt, remember that there are experienced practitioners available who will specialize in many forms of natural medicine, not least the growing army of vets trained in homeopathy and phytotherapy (the medicinal use of plants).

One example of an integrated approach to healing is that of treating a respiratory condition. You can begin treatment with energy therapy in order to help to revitalize the body, raise energy levels and encourage the body to begin to heal itself. You could also feed herbs like Garlic to help fight any infection that may be present, or Marshmallow to clear and soothe the airways, and deal with any irritation that may be either attributed to the problem or exacerbating it, such as an allergy. It is simple enough to combine both healing and herbs with a practical daily routine to help the animal regain fitness, by combining plenty of rest with a little light, regular exercise and a nutritious diet. These measures alone will often be sufficient to promote healing and bring the body back to health. Alternatively, you could introduce a blend of essential oils like Eucalyptus and Lemon, that can be used externally to help to clear and soothe the airways and ease the breathing. In this instance an oil blend could be of particular benefit during the animal's rest or sleep periods. You may find that a homeopathic Bach flower remedy is more suitable (such as Oak, to give strength, or Olive, for use at times of exhaustion), or you may wish to work with an appropriate crystal such as Quartz, to boost healing.

Where you are working to heal a stress-related behavioural issue, for example, you may wish to feed a combination of herbs that have calming, stabilizing or mildly sedative properties, such as Valerian and Camomile, which can help to promote relaxation and release fear. You could also use a deeply relaxing essential oil like Vetiver or Lavender to help to keep you and your pet calm; or you could administer a homeopathic Bach Flower remedy such as White Chestnut (to ease racing thoughts) as an aid to clearing mental or emotional negativity.

THE ENERGY OF VIBRATIONAL MEDICINE

Natural 'medicines' such as herbs, oils, flower remedies (all of which are, of course, different forms of plant) and crystals are known as vibrational or energy medicines. This is because they are thought to work on an energetic level, in much the same way as using simply energy on its own. The theory behind energy medicines is that they can work in one of several ways; either to match a vibration (or frequency) of energy within the body to boost it, so throwing off a negative condition; to introduce a vibration of energy that the body needs to help combat a particular condition; or to provide the opposite energetic force to that of the sickness, thus counteracting it. Such remedies can be thought of as energetic 'keys' to unlocking the healing process and providing a means of energetic shift and release. I recommend the use of vibrational medicines, obviously with the appropriate care, as I find them to be extremely useful energy 'tools' if used in this way.

Although energy medicines incorporate some of the oldest and most natural of remedies known to man, much of the knowledge behind their use has been lost. There is much to be done today to make up for this and to rediscover the

> 'Natural 'medicines' such as herbs, oils, flower remedies ... and crystals are known as vibrational or energy medicines... Such remedies can be thought of as energetic 'keys' to unlocking the healing process and providing a means of energetic shift and release.'

full benefits to be gained in working with them. Modern man is also in a better position than ever to uncover the 'why's and 'wherefores' of how these remedies work on the mind and body.

Homeopathic medicine, for example, though widely used and available, is still in many ways a mystery to us. The fact that the potency of each remedy increases the more dilute it becomes, is thought to be somehow related to the energetic imprint of the original, active ingredient. The interaction of homeopathic remedies with the body holds other secrets that have yet to come to light. It may be possible that the oft-maligned deactivation of the remedy that occurs on contact with the skin may be due simply to absorption of the energetic frequency of that remedy. Many other vibrational medicines can help to heal simply on coming into contact with the body (or the energy field of the body). A remedy on the right energetic frequency can be most effective in this way, and this can be tested for using kinesiology.

Kinesiology is a simple way to check whether the substance you are testing, maybe a remedy or a food, has a positive or negative effect on the energy of the body. With people, you can simply ask the person you are testing to hold out his or her arm at right angles to the body (horizontally) and keep it firm, but relaxed. Gently press the hand, just for a moment, to establish the natural strength of the body's energy – it may barely move (strong energy); it may dip slightly (OK); or it may drop (very low energy). The standard response is a slight dip. Then, keeping your pressures on the subject's hand uniform as you test, ask the person to hold, with the other hand, a food or substance that has a negative effect upon them – they might be allergic to it. If you test again, you will find that the arm drops – showing that the substance you are testing weakens the person's energy. Substances having a positive effect on the energy will enhance the individual's energy, and so the resistance of the subject's arm to pressure will be greater – there will be little, if any, 'dip' as you test.

You can test animals in the same way, but you need to use a person as a 'surrogate' – in other words, have the person maintain contact with the animal with one hand, and use the other arm to test with. Introduce substances to the animal by touching them against the animal's body, tucking them under the collar or even placing a co-operative paw on the substance! The practice of kinesiology has many uses and has echoes of the old children's custom of holding buttercups to the throat to see if one 'needs' or 'likes' butter.

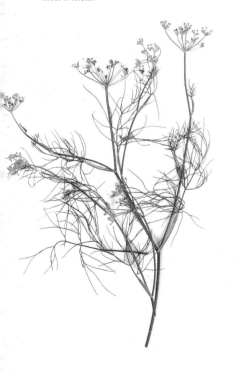

Fennel *(Foeniculum vulgare)* is excellent for assisting digestion and can be added to food. Some dogs and cats will eat it fresh after a meal.

The idea of efficacy of a remedy upon contact with the body is one that has been practised since time immemorial. Many cultures use amulets, which are thought to bestow the wearer with therapeutic properties, as a form of contact medicine. Amulets are worn by people, as well as being used to adorn all kinds of animals, and are found among ancient burial goods worldwide. They can be made from natural materials like plants, metals and stones, the relics from animals such as bones, teeth and feathers, and often include an element of colour. The composition of each amulet will vary according to its purpose and the elemental properties that the wearer needs. For example, a dog suffering injuries following a hostile encounter would be given an amulet for healing. This could be made from a turquoise stone, its copper content used to promote healing of the body; the feather of an eagle, to promote strength and courage in the face of adversity; and a sprig of a cleansing, tonic or anti-bacterial herb.

Natural medicines used in this way begin to have echoes of magic and indeed, the origin of much so-called 'magical' ritual is in the strength of nature and the many and varied energetic properties of natural ingredients. It is likely that many of the people who were once persecuted for being witches would be today's

Below. Using a human subject to test the horse's energy level. This technique – kinesiology – is a very useful tool to discover whether a particular food or a remedy has a positive or a negative effect on the animal you are treating.

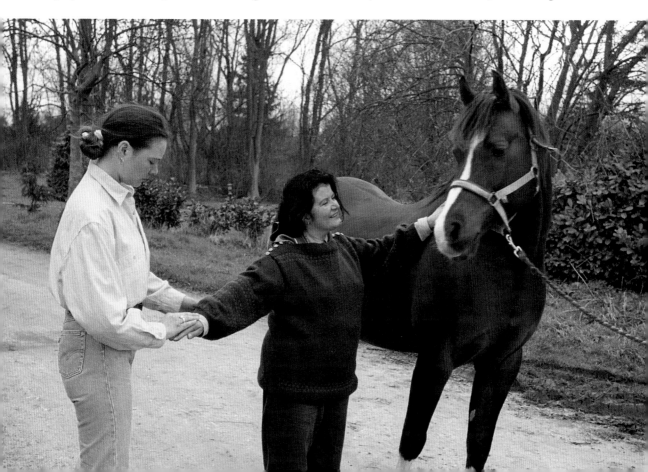

herbalists and healers. The psychologist Jung placed great importance on the negative view and even fear that some men have of women who are ' in touch with the forces of nature'. The 'spells' witches cast are primarily a manifestation of energy by intent and the projection of energy via objects is well known in this kind of work.

Today's crystal healers work primarily by boosting the energetic properties of stones with healing energy. The idea of investing an object with energy, be it for healing or any other aim, is far from being an old wives' tale – just think of sending someone a card or giving them a gift to say, 'I love you', 'Congratulations', 'Hi', or 'Sorry'!

THE BODY'S ENERGY CENTRES

Crystals, oils and other energy therapies are also powerful aids to the healing process when used in conjunction with the seven main chakras or energy centres of the body. I have heard, within the healing community, arguments that animals (but not including humans) don't have chakras, nor their own souls. Anyone who lives closely with animals will know that they clearly do have their own essential energy or soul. Those who are sensitive to energy will also tell you that animals certainly have energy centres within the physical body and energy field. If they had no energy centres it follows that they would also have no meridians or energy pathways – so acupuncture would not work for them, and it clearly does.

This kind of view, seeing humans as somehow above or superior to other animals, is a biblical one which pervades much of modern society. It is, however, incredibly limited and denies the huge richness in variation of forms of life and their capabilities. Other animals often display far more altruistic behaviour than do humans and work together for the greater good in a highly synchronistic way. Our own species is intent on wrecking its environment, waging war, inflicting all kinds of hardship upon its members and competing for resources which are fast running out! Compare this with dolphins, whose sensitivity to energies of all kinds gives them the ability to heal on a profoundly deep level, and who continue to offer help and friendship to mankind in the face of the atrocities we have inflicted upon them! Of course, this paints a negative picture of humanity – but it's a humbling view. The other point is that humans have the ability to make a choice. A large proportion of mankind is well aware of the rights and wrongs of its behaviour and yet government and individuals persist in the same old ways largely for individual gain and gratification, as well as to maintain a society based on consumerism.

With this in mind, I was once asked, 'Do horses have energy centres? What use is the crown chakra (the energy centre at the top of the head) to a horse?' My answer is that yes, all animals have energy centres. It is my experience that certain chakras are more important to and better developed in different species, in other words they are more involved in the animals' experiences than others. I am more aware of the strength of certain energy centres for different animals, as well as the distinction between them for various species. I have found that the more complex the animal, the more complex its energy makeup – so I have found distinct, strong energy centres in horses, less obvious in dogs and cats, and quite indistinct in say, rabbits. It's not so much a question of 'what use the chakras are' to the animal, it is a question of how the chakras are involved in the animal's life. The crown chakra, for example, is concerned with energetic input from outside. Such input comes from what most of us would term the 'source' of energy, so what this chakra is really about is our essence or soul, being connected with our source. So, the 'use' or function of an energy centre here, for the horse, is to receive the kind of input that affects the pattern of his life.

Such guidance for animals comes in a very instinctive way; a direct influence of behaviour through an awareness of something they experience the need to do, for example. In this way they influence the responses, behaviour and experiences of the humans (and other animals) that they are in contact with. Our own guidance or teaching in life comes in the form that we are most open to and for many people, this will be through their animals. So, for a horse who behaves in a certain way, this can lead to the person he influences learning all kinds of new things as a necessary reaction to that. I suspect that all of you reading this book have been influenced to do so by something that your animals have done or experienced! During my workshops or my lectures, I always ask: 'How many of you would be here if not for your pet?' Rarely is a hand raised. Dogs so fearful that they cannot be left alone, aggressive cats which nothing seems to calm, are just the animals who push their owners to seek new ways to help them.

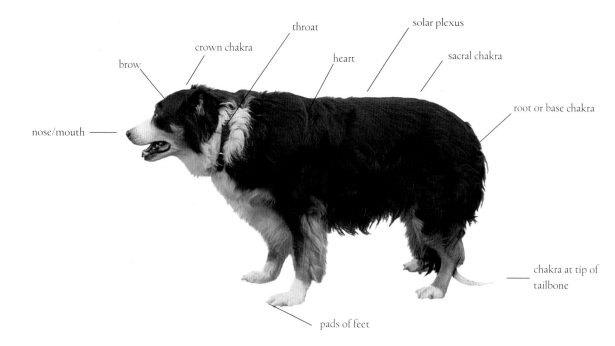

brow

crown chakra

throat

heart

solar plexus

sacral chakra

root or base chakra

nose/mouth

chakra at tip of tailbone

pads of feet

Above. Animals have their energy centres in a similar location to humans, with the addition of an energy centre or chakra at the tip of the tailbone. Remember: chakras are not a physical 'spot' on the body, but are many-dimensional.

Opposite page. Gem, a rescued guinea pig with a lucky escape.

The chakras each have a slightly different range of frequency of energy. Each frequency or energetic pattern is influenced by and corresponds to energies within the individual that can be translated as thought and manifested as behaviour. Conversely, behaviours and thoughts can influence the energy of the chakras relating to those frequencies, causing blockages or stagnation of energy and thus, physical dis-ease (or negative physical condition). The frequencies of the chakras can be matched or reproduced by the energetic frequencies of different colours, notes of music, and elemental materials such as stones, metals, and plants. Plants can also be used in forms such as oil, homeopathic remedies, and herbs or food to match or reproduce these frequencies. Each method can thus be used therapeutically to help to shift the energy surrounding physical dis-ease or behavioural patterns related to particular chakras. In reality, many animals' issues are related to root chakra stagnation or blockage.

It would take another book to go into depth about the chakras each animal has, the energies involved with each chakra and the issues related to this for various species of animal; as well as to relate each remedy within every different kind of vibrational therapy to the chakra it is relevant to. There are books detailing the therapeutic use of essential oils with the chakras, of music, colour and of course, crystals and I would encourage those interested to study them.

The negative conditions, both physical and behavioural, that animals of all kinds suffer are largely related to blockages of energy around the root chakra. This is the energy centre that resonates to 'feelings' or frequencies of energy related to basic, instinctual needs – such as food, shelter, reproduction and maintaining territory. In very simple terms, the kind of experience that can cause an energetic blockage in this area is likely to be one related to extreme fear: of not having enough food, of being hurt or in deadly danger, for example. I generally think of the root chakra as located at the base of an animal's tail, where it meets the body. Sometimes, I feel similar energies right at the end of the tail – cats and some dogs love having the tip of their tail gently held during a healing treatment. It is a good idea to concentrate on the tail area of any animal suffering stress or behavioural trauma, in particular. All forms of healing work to clear and boost the energy flow of the body, so the chakras are an important factor in establishing and maintaining that flow.

My aim in the next chapter is to give some guidelines for several of the more popular forms of self-help therapy which I have used, and which you can experiment with to help heal your pet, alongside giving him healing energy. There are many excellent and detailed books on all of these therapies for human use, and some for animals, too, so I will leave the detail to the specialists and simply give some basic information, based on my own experience, that you can start out with.

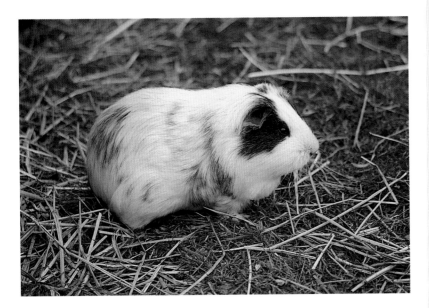

Rescue for Gem

Gem is a black and white guinea pig owned by a family with three children: Natalie, Charlotte and George. Gem was out playing in the garden with the children one day, but they were unaware that the family dog, Caspar, was loose, instead of safe in his run. Caspar came to investigate the fun and decided that Gem looked like a great game. He jumped on her, batting her around with his feet as if she were a toy, while she squeaked in panic and the children desperately tried to get Caspar to stop.

Natalie ran and fetched her mother, who grabbed Caspar and got him to settle down. But it looked like as if help had come too late for Gem. Shocked and battered, she was a limp little animal who looked ready to give up. Once Caspar was safely shut in, Sharon, Natalie's mother, gently picked up Gem and took her inside to see what could be done. The children were clearly upset, and their mother, who had learned healing just the week before, found she had to comfort the children first in order to give Gem any peace – the children were all given a good dose of Bach Flower Rescue Remedy. Sharon then held Gem and worked on her. There were no signs of bleeding or cuts, but she seemed to be deeply shocked. After some fifteen minutes, Gem began to move around a little. Sharon decided it was safe to take her to the vet and that she was strong enough to travel. She kept Gem in her lap during the car journey and felt her gradually getting stronger and calmer.

By the time they reached the surgery, Gem appeared to have returned to normal, and luckily, on examination, it was revealed that she had escaped serious injury. Sharon felt that Gem had been in such deep shock when she found her that, had she got to her much later, Gem would never have survived. She continued to treat Gem for the next couple of weeks to make sure she was back on form.

ENERGY MEDICINE FOR ANIMALS

HERBAL REMEDIES

Where an imbalance in nutrition may have been involved in bringing about the presenting problem that your pet is suffering from, or where introducing nutritional factors could help to alleviate the symptoms of a condition, I tend to advise the use of herbs as part of an animal's diet. Herbs are the original source of the active ingredients of many synthetic drugs and thus can be considered as nature's own 'medicine'. If you read an old herbal reference book like Culpeper's, you will be astonished at the vague way in which he describes many plants that you might never even have heard of, let alone seen, as 'so well-known as not to need description'. This is a symptom of the change in our lifestyle during the last couple of centuries.

At one time, we all grew or had access to a wide variety of medicinal plants and, if we couldn't lay our hands on what we wanted, a short walk and we could easily have identified and found the herb we needed. Sadly, many herbs have become unfashionable in the garden in favour of cultivated flowers. Many herbs, often being unspectacular in appearance, were removed from the garden and dismissed as a weed, and in this way, we have lost many valuable plants that used to grow in abundance.

Feeding a herb internally is a fast, effective and direct method of administering a new energetic vibration, or gently boosting an energetic vibration within the body. As our animals are rarely in a position to seek the herbs they might require to help maintain their own health, it is up to us to make what they might need available. I use the term 'make available' because I believe that animals, with their acute senses and synchronicity with their own bodies and nature, should be given as much choice in their own healing as possible. Administering a herb that an animal doesn't want to eat is rarely beneficial. My experience is that most animals will eat and can be fed small doses of herbs quite safely, and that they really enjoy them, but if in doubt, consult an expert.

ADMINISTRATION AND DOSAGE

Fresh herbs. Any herb you gather from the wild should be taken from as clean and fresh a source as possible – not sprayed, fertilized or otherwise tampered with. Most herbs that you gather can be fed fresh, but any with hairy stems or leaves should be wilted for a couple of hours before offering them to your pet, along with his normal meal. If you are administering a therapeutic dose, you can chop them manually or in a blender to make a paste. You can first test your animal's response by offering a little to be licked off your hand, and then add the paste to the feed. Fresh herbs can be offered ad-lib or fed chopped at up to 15g (approx. 3–5 teaspoons) per day for large dogs like labradors, decreasing the dosage for smaller animals to around 7g (2 teaspoons) for cats.

Dried herbs. Many herbs are available singly in dried form as a good second choice to fresh supplies, and the dosage of the active ingredients will be higher per weight fed, due to the lack of water. Try to avoid herbs that have been over-processed or that have been sitting in a shop for a long time. Dried herbs can be fed at 5-10g (roughly 1–3 teaspoons) per day in the feed.

DECOCTION

You can make a decoction of fresh or dried plants by adding up to 100g (4oz) of fresh herb to a 600ml (1 pint) of water (ideally spring water). Bring quickly to the boil, turn off the heat and allow to steep. Use the decoction the same day or keep in a fridge for up to a week. Feed 15ml (1 tablespoon) of the decoction at a time or use externally. Decoctions can be used for dressings, or adding to a pre-prepared lotion or cream, such as Bach Flower Rescue Cream, or other natural preparations.

As with all natural therapies, only use herbs for as long as a condition indicates it. When your pet chooses not to take the herbs any longer, or the condition clears up, stop using the preparation.

FAVOURITE HERBS FOR PETS

Cleavers or Goosegrass *Galium aparine* (see page 79): This has a number of other names according to where you live, and is often called 'Sweethearts' because of the little hairs that make the seeds stick together (and to anything

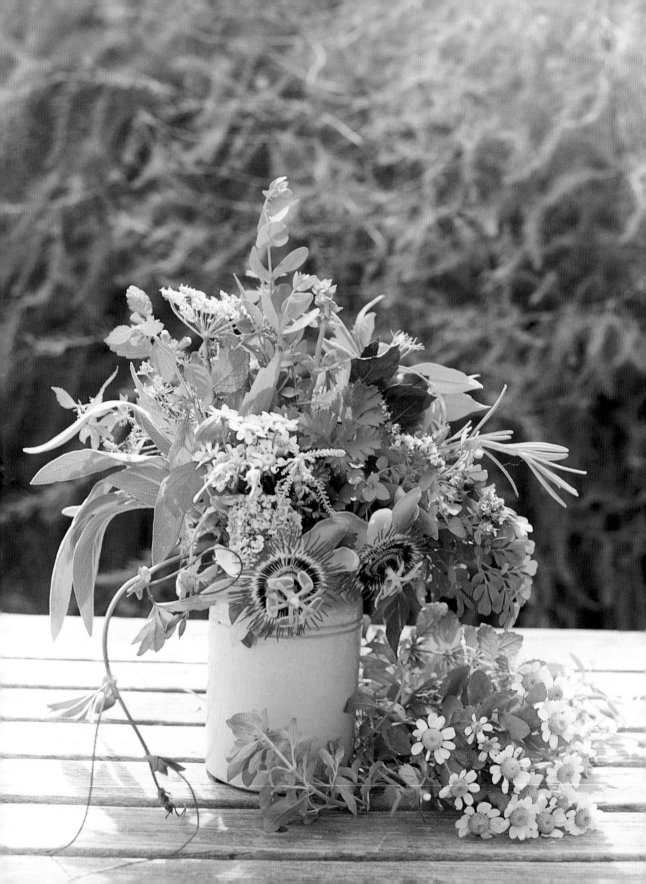

else!). It grows in fields and hedgerows, almost all year round and is generally known as a weed. You can pick handfuls of it fresh and offer it to your dog or cat (dogs often eat it if they can find it whilst out walking), or dry it and process for use later. This is one plant you won't be able to buy dried, as far as I know, from suppliers. It has so many uses that I consider it an essential; it is wonderful for boosting immunity and in all cases of infection. The high silica content makes it invaluable for conditions involving bones, hair and teeth, and it can be used externally to encourage expulsion of infected material. Use the whole plant.

Nettle There are many different kinds of Nettle, but the common stinging nettle, *Urtica dioica,* is abundant everywhere. Nettles are extremely high in vitamins (particularly vitamin C) and iron, as well as having gently diuretic qualities. They can be fed wherever the system needs 'cleaning'; for animals with skin conditions, joint problems, and toxins in the system. You'll need to wear gardening gloves to avoid being stung. Cut the stems and wilt them before offering to your pet, to let the sting go off. Some animals will prefer them gently cooked in water and will eat them like a vegetable. If you're drying Nettles, only use the leaves; you can also buy dried Nettle leaves from good herbalists.

Dandelion *Taraxacum officinale*: This plant has the effect of balancing fluid, so it works both as a diuretic and an electrolyte according to the body's needs. Another 'cleansing' herb, you can feed the root, which is quite strong and has a powerful effect, or the leaves, which are more gentle. Very useful for any problems where the body is not expelling toxins adequately. When I was a child we always gathered Dandelion leaves for our rabbits and tortoises, who loved them. The herb, in its fresh and dry state, is illustrated on page 83.

Garlic *Allium sativum*: The most commonly fed herb, but ideally should be given at the rate of one fresh crushed clove per day rather than the processed form. This is the great natural antibiotic and helps to deal with infection of all kinds, from bronchial and viral to invasive external infections. Due to its purifying action it is helpful for all kinds of skin conditions and aids digestion. It is strongly anti-parasitic so repels insects and internal worms. Use the whole clove and feed the fresh growing leaves.

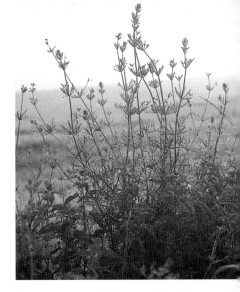

Above: Cleavers (*Galium aparine*). A high silica content makes this plant invaluable for treating a variety of ailments.

Opposite page. A selection of medicinal herbs collected in the garden and in the hedgerows. They should be put in water immediately and used as quickly as possible after picking.

Below. White Deadnettle (*Lamium album*) is a digestive and is also useful for conditions affecting the urinary tract.

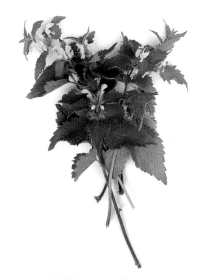

Camomile *Chamaemelum nobile* (see page 10): Camomile grows wild in many countries and is the best first recourse for all kinds of tension-related issues. I also use it externally to soothe skin and encourage healing. I generally feed it as part of any mixture where nerves may be exacerbating, or related to, the presenting condition. Use both flowers and leaves.

Meadowsweet *Filipendula ulmaria* (see page 82): You can gather Meadowsweet from the wild or buy it dried. I prefer to use it dried, both for external and internal use, as it is only the flowers and leaves that are useful. It contains salicylic acid, the active ingredient isolated and manufactured into aspirin. It has a wide variety of uses from healing internal bleeding and ulcers (unlike synthetic aspirin, which can have the opposite effect), as well as for coughs, and to aid digestion and reduce scouring. It also helps pain due to inflammation and heat.

Comfrey *Symphytum officinale* (see page 83): Comfrey grows wild everywhere and used to be a favourite garden plant. It was once reputed as a heal-all and is ideal for external use on wounds and for any skin condition when made into a paste. It is anti-inflammatory, hence its use for joint problems such as arthritis, and it can also be given for coughs. Use the whole plant, but wilt before feeding fresh to let the hairs on the leaves settle.

Marigold *Calendula officinalis* (see page 83): Marigold petals are one of my favourite stand-bys for everything from healing external skin conditions to digestive disorders. Ideal for skin problems. Only the flowers are used for treatment, both externally and internally. Lots of cats and dogs will eat fresh Marigold flowers if you have them growing in the garden.

Valerian *Valeriana officinalis* (see page 83): A most calming, sedative herb, which should be fed in limited quantity. You can find it growing wild but it is easier to handle bought dry as you will only use the roots. Beware, because it smells pretty unpleasant! It is ideal for nervous animals and is slightly laxative. It should not be used in excess; feed only 5g (1–2 teaspoons) daily to start with.

Marshmallow *Althaea officinalis* (see page 46): You can find or grow Marshmallow or buy it dried. It is very syrupy when blended with liquid so is ideal for coughs of all kinds and as a generally soothing treatment for gastric complaints and inflammation elsewhere in the body. You can use it as an ointment or dressing externally and make it into a lovely soothing milk drink for yourself.

Sage *Salvia officinalis* (see page 83): Sage is my favourite hormonal balancer because it doesn't over-stimulate. It is also a natural antibiotic so, when combined with Garlic, is ideal for any sort of infection. Many animals thrive on Sage and it can give animals struggling with hormonal issues a whole new lease of life. Feed a few fresh leaves or up to 10g (3 teaspoons) dry herb daily for larger animals.

Devils Claw *Arpagopythum procumbens*: Available only in pre-prepared form, it is the best tonic I know for inflammatory issues like arthritis, which affect so many pets, particularly in the winter. Always a viable option for animals suffering from any kind of inflammation.

BEST HERBAL BLENDS

The herbal blends included here are ones I regularly make up for use as dry blends to be fed as part of treatment programmes. Mix the ingredients in equal quantities.

◆ For any lymphatic, immune or other condition that needs cleansing and boosting: Cleavers, Nettle, Dandelion and Garlic (all detailed above).

◆ Gastric problems and skin complaints: Cleavers, Meadowsweet and Marigold, with the addition of Camomile where necessary for stress reduction (all detailed above).

◆ For tension: Valerian, Vervain *Verbena officinalis* (dried leaves), Hops (buy dried heads) and Camomile or Poppy seeds.

◆ For scurf or skin problems: Nettle, Dandelion, Marigold, Garlic (all detailed above).

◆ Joint problems: Comfrey, Meadowsweet or Devil's Claw (all detailed above).

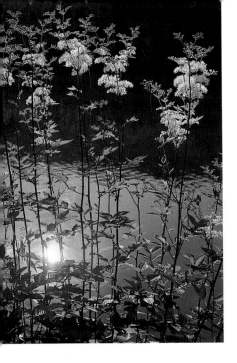

◆ For scour: Meadowsweet, Slippery Elm *Ulmus rubra* (in powder form), Yarrow *Achillea millefolium* (available as a prepared dried herb).

◆ For constipation: Nettles, Valerian, Dandelion, Fennel (*Foeniculum officinalis,* see page 70).

◆ For aggressive behaviour: Sage, Valerian, Camomile, Passionflower *Passiflora incarnata* (available as a dried herb or tincture).

◆ To stimulate: Garlic, Cleavers, Mint (*Mentha*), Fennel, Rosemary (*Rosmarinus officinalis*). (The latter three herbs can be bought in dried form; the other two are detailed above.)

◆ For coughs: Garlic, Meadowsweet, Marshmallow, Mint (see above).

◆ As a diuretic: Dandelion, Nettle (as detailed above).

Meadowsweet *(Filipendula ulmaria)* is high in salicylic acid, a natural pain-relief agent from which aspirin is derived.

BACH FLOWER REMEDIES

Bach remedies are one of a wide variety of off-the-shelf homeopathic preparations that you can buy from any chemist or health food store. Like most preparations, they have been designed and marketed for human administration, but unlike many other remedies, these are totally safe when given to animals – even if you're a beginner (refer to dosage guidelines on page 85).

Below. The whole range of Bach remedies

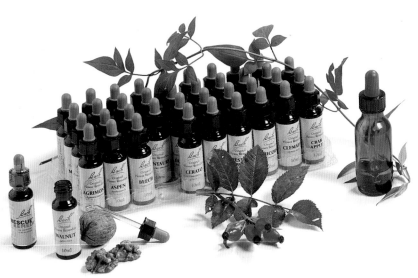

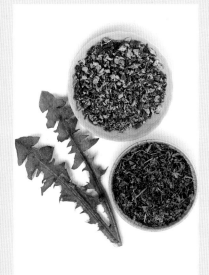

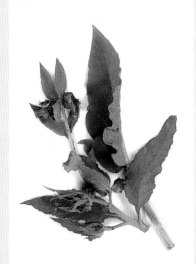

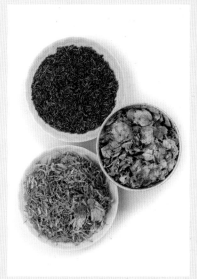

Fresh Dandelion leaves are an effective diuretic. The dry root, shown on the top right of the picture, is a powerful 'cleansing' agent which helps the body expelling toxins. The leaves can also be given dry (bottom right of picture).

Comfrey is easy to find around the countryside. It is a good herb for wounds and a variety of skin conditions. It is also effective for joint complaints such as arthritis.

Top. Caraway seeds promote a healthy appetite and are also digestive. Left. Marigold petals (see page 80) also good for ear, nose and throat problems. Hops, on the right, are digestive, also help emotional problems due to stress.

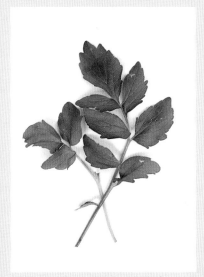

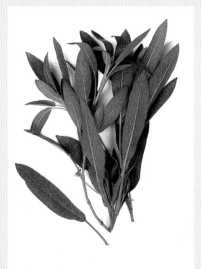

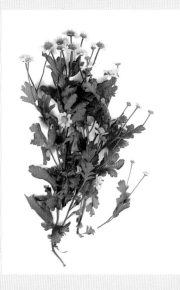

Valerian. The root of the plant is used and you may find easier to use in its dry state. See page 80 for advice on how to administer it.

Fresh Sage (see page 81). Sage is also excellent for digestion and liver complaints as well as for nervous stressed conditions.

Feverfew. For centuries this plant was the traditional way of relieving fever. The leaves can be made into a tea or chopped up on food.

Bach remedies were formulated in the 1930s by former Harley Street doctor, Edward Bach. There are thirty-eight separate remedies made from the distilled roots, flowers and leaves of plants, which have been diluted to a homeopathic level and then preserved in brandy. They are designed for home use as well as by trained therapists, and the worst that happens if you administer the wrong remedy is that it simply doesn't work.

The remedies number among therapies known as 'vibrational', because the energetic pattern of each remedy matches, introduces or enhances a vibration to or within the body to which they are administered. In this way, the remedies work on the mental or behavioural issues behind what have often become physical conditions. So, you can use them to treat behavioural or emotional problems in your animals (and yourself) as well as the behavioural causes behind physical disease – for example, stress causing low immunity and thus susceptibility to viral infection. It's important to remember, though, that there may be an underlying cause behind your pets' problems, which needs to be addressed. In other words, it's all very well giving a tense animal a remedy to relax him, but for a truly holistic, thorough approach, you should look at other factors that may be making him tense.

FAVOURITE BACH REMEDIES FOR PETS

Rescue Remedy: Probably the best-known Bach remedy is Rescue Remedy, which is a blend of several individual flower remedies known to be particularly effective for shock and trauma. It is a great standby for the first-aid kit and I advise people to take it themselves and to give it to their pets in cases of accident, injury, in sickness such as colic, and after giving birth. It has a calming effect on humans and animals who are stressed, anxious or in a state of panic.

Walnut: Walnut is ideal to keep around for times of change – which, let's face it, is often what life is all about. Walnut can help animals who have changed owners or moved house, or whose circumstances are otherwise altered, such as when a new pet joins the family.

Vervain: Vervain is for counteracting tension and anxiety, so is ideal for animals who have anxiety-related behavioural issues. It's also a useful long-term aid where animals are particularly nervy or highly strung.

Aspen, Mimulus, Rock Rose: These are all remedies for fear – Aspen for vague fears: Mimulus for fears related to a real event or object: and Rock Rose for terror. Choose the appropriate remedy for animals who are afraid of things like cats of dogs, traffic, loud noises...the list is endless.

Elm, Larch: These remedies are beneficial to pets who react badly when left alone.

Olive: This is a great remedy to give to convalescing pets. It helps to give a lift mentally and rally flagging spirits that feel totally exhausted.

Chestnut Bud, Honeysuckle: Both are handy in situations where you are trying to retrain a pet or teach him something new. Honeysuckle helps the mind to move forward by letting go of the past, so that old habits can be released and new ways learned. Chestnut Bud helps to facilitate learning and is the remedy for letting go of past mistakes.

BLENDING YOUR OWN BACH REMEDIES

You can blend anything up to seven remedies together to form an individual remedy for yourself or your pet, according to the circumstances and the needs of the individual being treated. If you are uncertain which to choose, go for one to start with and then add another remedy to see if it has the desired effect, rather than using a complex blend and not knowing which remedy works and which doesn't. Use two to four drops of each remedy you want to blend in 75ml (5 tablespoons) of spring water.

DOSAGE GUIDELINES FOR BACH FLOWER REMEDIES

Two to four drops of the chosen remedy (or blend) can be added to your pet's drinking water four times a day. For very small animals just give two drops twice daily. You can also give the remedy directly from the droppers on the top of the bottle, but beware because the dropper tubes are made of glass. You will also be giving the remedy undiluted, which will give your pet a direct shot of the alcohol (brandy) that the remedy is preserved in, and alcohol for pets is hardly natural or advisable. You can add the remedies to your pet's feed but, as with any homeopathic preparation, once they are in contact with a substance their effect is absorbed, so it is best to give them as directly to the animal as

Neil has a tank where he keeps five cold-water fish that he took over from friends. Earlier this year, one of his chums turned up on the doorstep with a stunning little fish, bright orange in colour and with a wonderful sweeping tail. The boy had won the fish at a fair but didn't have a tank, so he thought Neil would like to keep him. Neil was really impressed with the new fish and called him Fizz. For the first couple of days, Fizz seemed to settle well in his new environment.

Sadly, fish that are won at fairs have often been moved around quite a lot and gone through several changes of water and environment. All of this can affect their health to such a degree that they often don't survive the ordeal. After three days, Neil noticed the tell-tale signs that Fizz was far from well. He was bobbing about near the surface, gulping for air, had stopped eating and was losing his balance. As the day went on, Fizz seemed to get worse and Neil, having seen this happen many times before, expected the fish to die.

That day, I was treating Neil's sisters dog, and she jokingly asked if I could do anything for Fizz. I honestly had no idea but I knew from experience that fish are really fragile. Still, we felt it couldn't do any harm to give it a try. I put my hands in the water around where Fizz was and just let the energy come through. After I'd done all I felt I could do, I left in the tank a couple of amethyst crystals that I had charged up with energy, to act like a healing 'battery' for the fish. That evening and for a few more days I sent Fizz some healing.

With a previous case I hadn't treated the fish but had 'charged up' crystals before putting them in the water. That fish hadn't survived, so I was delighted when Neil said shortly afterwards that Fizz had fully recovered. Perhaps we just got to him in time, or he was especially tough, but he certainly surprised us.

possible. People, on the other hand, should take four drops either directly under the tongue or in a glass of water, four times a day.

CRYSTAL THERAPY FOR BALANCE AND HARMONY

Whether you realize it or not, crystals are all around us every day of our lives. Almost everyone has a ring with a stone in it or a watch with a quartz crystal inside. Because of their capacity to store and conduct energetic charges, crystals are included in all kinds of electrical equipment – so there's nothing strange or outlandish about them. Crystal therapy is the most beautiful and the safest therapy that you can try out for yourself at home.

Crystals are also colourful and wonderful to look at and to hold, which is therapeutic in itself. The colour that our eyes see is the colour of light that a stone reflects – so a red crystal absorbs every other colour within the spectrum except red light. The colour reflected depends upon the atomic structure of the crystal, giving each crystal it's own atomic vibrational frequency. You can think of the frequency of crystals like notes of music within the octave (the octave and light spectrum being similar natural arrangements – as the seven main chakras are said to be). Each crystal of the same basic colour can be thought of as having a different 'pitch' of the same 'note' or frequency, like the idea of a low C or a high C. Then, due to its structure, each crystal of that 'pitch' has a different 'tone' – like the difference between a sharp, ringing note and a soft, muted one. Crystals do, in fact, resonate to sound but sadly it is way above the range of frequency of human hearing. I'm not so sure that it's above the range of animals' hearing, though.

The frequency of vibration of each crystal matches a frequency of vibration within the body, and in some cases introduces a new one that the body can absorb – this includes both the physical body and the energy body or aura. The idea of crystal therapy, then, can be likened to tuning a piano – finding the duff notes (or blocks and kinks in energy) in the body and using a crystal to increase or boost the resonation or vibration of energy, and tune up the body. Maybe this is where the term 'being in harmony' or 'being in tune' comes from.

CHOOSING AND USING CRYSTALS

Crystals are chosen and used for their vibrational frequencies, and the effect this has on the physical and energy body that they are applied to. This is why stones are often said to 'signify' certain things – for example a stone 'for love' vibrates

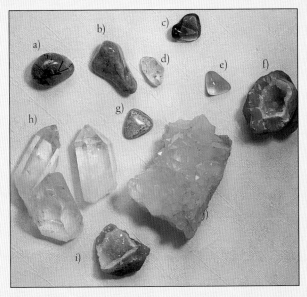

a) Tourmaline in
   Quartz
b) Rhodonite
c) Smoky Quartz

d) Herkimer
   Diamond
e) pink Fluorite
f) geode

g) Rhodocrosite
h) Quartz points
i) geode
j) Quartz cluster

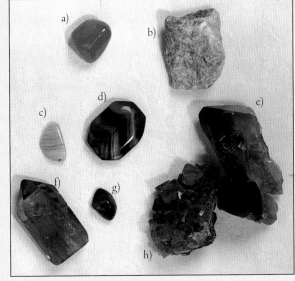

a) Agate
b) Lepidolite
c) Blue Lace Agate

d) Fluorite
e) Amethyst
   points
f) Ametrine

g) Watermelon
   Tourmaline
h) Amethyst cluster

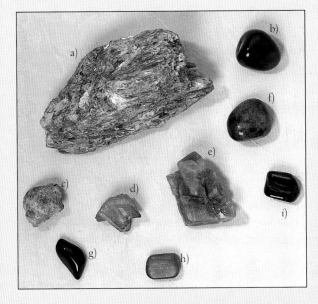

a) Kyanite
b) Agate
c) Azurite

d) Aqua Aura
e) blue Calcite
f) Sodalite

g) blue Tigers Eye
h) Lapiz lazuli
i) blue Tigers Eye

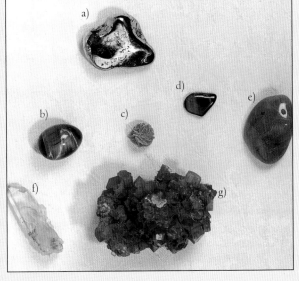

a) Copper
b) Tigers Eye
c) Selenite (gypsum)

d) red Tigers Eye
e) rutilated Quartz
f) Citrine

g) Aragonite

at the frequency of those 'feelings' or vibrations within the body, so the stone can increase or introduce that vibration or 'feeling' into the body. This also explains why people and animals are drawn to certain stones – because at some level, they need that energy amplified, boosted, or introduced, and enjoy the feeling this brings. Animals are particularly quick to choose the crystals they like or need, perhaps because, with their more sensitive hearing, they can actually pick up far more of the total energy picture of a given stone. Generally speaking, if your pet is drawn to a specific stone, that's the one he needs. Animals can also be given the choice from a variety laid in front of them – dogs in particular are quite definite about their choices, and often steal what they want.

WHICH CRYSTAL?

There are hundreds of different rocks and minerals that have therapeutic effects. In line with most vibrational therapies, crystals do not even have to touch the physical body in order to have an appreciable effect. They can be used anywhere – placed in the home or the stable or stall, kennel, cage, hutch, run or fish tank – anywhere they can't be swallowed by an inquisitive animal. Crystals can also be tied to collars, placed under bandages, tied to a horse's tack, or stitched into the corners of blankets, beds and rugs. Large crystals can be left in your pet's water-dish. Crystals can be made into elixirs with spring water for animals to drink, and I often use them in Bach remedies and essential oil blends to add their own healing properties. Crystals can also be directly applied to the skin singly or in groups as you treat with energy therapy. For truly beneficial effect, the crystal should be carried until it becomes apparent that your pet no longer needs it.

When you buy a crystal, don't buy it simply for its attractive colour, see how it feels to you. Sometimes, if it has been handled by lots of people, it may have picked up negative charges and need cleansing. The best way to cleanse most crystals is to place them outside in the sun for a few hours, leave them on a windowsill in the moonlight overnight, or rinse them with spring water. You can also cleanse and charge them up by holding them in your hands and giving them healing energy. Many people say that it is important to 'program' a crystal for the task you are using it for – I have never found this to be true. Just knowing what you want to use a stone for is enough to add your own intent to the positive charge of the stone.

FAVOURITE CRYSTALS FOR ANIMALS

The most commonly found, safe and easy to use crystals for healing are:

Clear Quartz: An excellent all-rounder, Quartz is the best stone to start out with as it amplifies healing energy and is great for clearing blockages. Its main function is to stimulate the body into self-healing. Use for any condition where the body needs help to heal.

Rose Quartz: A pink Quartz, which is very comforting, peaceful and balancing. Its main function is to transmit energy between people or animals in a relationship, so it's a good stone for pets who have come to a new owner, or if you leave your animals and go on holiday. Very good for people and animals who feel unloved or lack confidence in themselves.

Amethyst: A lavender-coloured Quartz, excellent for raising awareness and settling the temper. It is also said to be helpful to keep a large crystal in your pet's water, to reduce infections, parasites and insect invasions like mites. You can also use it as a base in a fish tank, which makes a beautiful feature as well as imparting its benefits to the tank's occupants.

Calcites: These soft stones come in many colours, and are particularly soothing and cleansing. They are very good for pain of all kinds, particularly in the joints. You can apply a stone directly to a pulled muscle or an ache of any kind, and on areas of inflamed or burnt skin (do clean the stone properly before using on another animal). Very good for pets with skin problems of all kinds.

Agates: Also in many colours, these are real worker-stones. In broad terms, they affect the stomach, so are grounding for nervous animals, for giving strength, and for finicky eaters.

Tigers Eye: in red, blue or gold, this is the stone for courage, willpower and clarity. Great for focusing animals who are unsure of themselves, perhaps when going to shows or just out into the world for the first few times.

Haematite: This is a very grounding stone, so not right for those who tend to feel 'low'. Suits animals with very scattered energy ('hyper' dogs and cats) as it centres the body and brings you back down to earth.

Citrine: a clear yellow Quartz, which works on the stomach area to reduce tension and on the mind to reduce confusion. It is also great for detoxification, so can be used as an elixir for convalescing pets to clear the system.

Labradorite: Blue or white, this is the most wonderful soothing, healing stone. It has a very calming influence on animals and people and brings light into the aura or energy field, encouraging healing.

Other stones that are very beneficial, but should be used with rather more care, include Lapis, Selenite, Turquoise, Moldavite, Herkimer Diamond, Fluorite and Aqua Aura. They are mostly employed by trained therapists. Lapis opens up your intuition, and can help working dogs, but only suits those with a calm nature. Selenite is really helpful for balancing the energy of people and animals, especially for epilepsy, but should really only be used by an experienced therapist as it has an extremely powerful effect, particularly on the brain. Turquoise is a good all-round healer due to its copper content, and is very uplifting for convalescing pets. Moldavite can be used in cases of severe depression, such as after the death of an owner, and pets with serious illness, especially in 'touch and go' or accident situations. Herkimer Diamond is again really a therapist's stone as it is a strong conductor of energy, so is powerful in healing sessions. Fluorite is very soothing, balancing and calming and is said to help repel colds and 'flu. Aqua Aura is another therapists's stone that can be helpful for pets with behavioural problems.

ESSENTIAL OILS

Essential oils have a myriad of complex energetic properties that are beneficial in introducing energy to the body of all species. They can be the key to unlocking all kinds of physical and behavioural tensions, giving you a way in to the animal's problems. Oils contain not only the vibrational pattern of the crystalline structure within the plants they are derived from, but also carry colour and scent, which are deep and profound stimuli to the brain. Use of scent can help to release and recharge all kinds of negative energy patterns quickly, painlessly and simply. This is of particular benefit to animals that, in their deepest states of distress, can accept the therapeutic properties of comforting scents – you don't even have to touch them.

GUIDELINES FOR USING OILS

It is vital to give animals the choice to work with you when offering oils. For large animals like horses or ponies and dogs, you can work quite safely with oils so long as you make certain you know which are safe to use and when. For cats and smaller animals, essential oils can prove too potent unless used very subtly, ideally just in the animal's home environment. Animals will make clear their interest in any given oil, as well as their lack of interest in it. Always offer an oil to the animal prior to administering it and as a true test of whether your pet needs it or not, offer the bottle, uncapped, to the animal's nose (hold it tightly in case he decides to try and take it) and let your pet tell you how he feels. The strongest positive response will be inhalation into both nostrils – thus carrying the aroma to both sides of the brain. (See picture on page 94.) Often, as a first treatment, this is enough for your pet and you will have to wait until later that

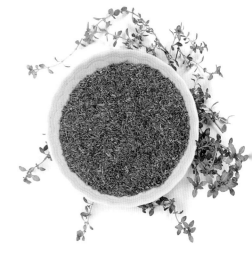

Dried and fresh Thyme (*Thymus vulgaris*). An oil is distilled from this plant which is a powerful antiseptic and a great expectorant. The oil is therefore ideal for treating chest infections.

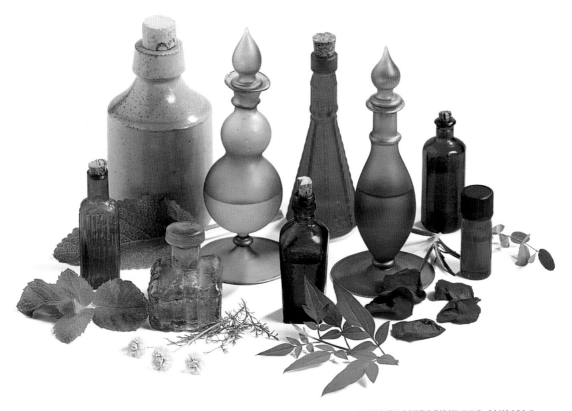

day to administer the oil again. Your pet will make his feelings equally clear when he has no further need for a particular oil. There is no point in saving what you have blended (a blend is a dilution of essential oil(s) in a carrier oil – see below) for another time, or using it up, as over-doing the treatment is unnecessary and unfair. As with all vibrational therapies, aroma can be a key to unlocking the door of many problems; particularly with animals that have been evasive of other therapies. It can often lead on to deeper issues that will then need to be addressed.

Many oils carry warnings that they should not be used during pregnancy, or neat on the skin, or internally. If in doubt, the simplest answer is don't. Tea-tree oil, in particular, should be used with care as it can cause short-term paralysis in dogs. Always consult a detailed text if you have any doubts.

DOSAGE AND ADMINISTRATION OF ESSENTIAL OILS

Internally: Dogs and some cats will be keen to lick neat essential oils either off the top of the bottle, from your hand, or the rim of their feed bowl. Never administer more than one neat drop per day in this way. I tend to only allow this in cases where the animal seems desperate to get to the oil, as I prefer to offer the oil in a blend – it's so much safer.

Externally: Oils can be applied by dabbing or spraying a blend on to your pet's, coat, collar, bowl, bed, blanket – in fact anywhere he has access to gentle inhalation. Fresh applications should be made both morning and evening or as required. Alternatively, you can use oils sparingly to give your pet a gentle massage twice a day, but be aware that he should not be allowed out into bright sunlight or hot weather directly afterwards, due to the risk of burning. I generally don't advise massage for anything other than large animals – and, besides, it can get quite messy. Some dogs and cats enjoy a mini-massage on the pads of their feet. Use your own judgment over external application and always under-use rather than over-apply. Proceed with care on pink skin, which is more sensitive, and maintain awareness of skin condition in case of allergic reaction. The only oil that can ever be applied neat to skin is Lavender.

BLENDING AND STORAGE OF OILS

There are many base oils for blending, but I choose either Sweet Almond, though it does have a slight scent of its own, or Grapeseed, which is least oily and least scented.

The dilutions at which you use various oils depend upon their pungency, but as a rough rule of thumb, I recommend 5 drops of essential oil in 15ml (one tablespoon) of carrier oil. Many of the small blending bottles which are sold for storage hold either 75ml (5 tablespoons), for which you will need 25-30 drops of essential oil; or 100ml (roughly 7 tablespoons), for which you will need approx 35 drops of essential oil. However many oils you blend, the total number of essential oil drops to carrier oil should be the same. A fresh oil has a shelf life of a couple of months in a plastic bottle, longer if stored in a dark glass bottle or jar with an airtight stopper, away from heat and light.

In terms of blending, experience and, obviously, your pet's choice will tell you what to do. However, as a general rule, keep groups of oils together such as sedative, stimulating and so on. Additional vibrational qualities can be added to an oil by the inclusion of fresh plant ingredients, crystals, or both. As with all vibrational medicines, experiment with using an integrated approach – for example, apply an oil blend to your hands before energy therapy treatment.

FAVOURITE OILS FOR PETS

Lavender is the quartz of essential oils! It has so many uses they are almost impossible to list. It will calm nervous animals, revive tired ones, heal wounds, keep away flies, and is even mildly stimulant to the immune system. It can be applied neat to scar tissue and healed wounds to encourage regrowth of healthy cells. A must, either on its own or as part of a blend.

Tea-tree oil is well known for its antiseptic and antibiotic properties, which can also be applied neat to wounds although it can sting. Do not use on a dog as Tea-tree can cause them temporary paralysis, and is so strong that it can cause discomfort to raw or sensitive skin. Very powerful, but use with care.

.**Clary Sage** is *the* hormonal balancer and, along with Geranium (very soothing and balancing), is indicated for use with animals that have either physical or behavioural problems related to hormone imbalance. It is also centring for scattered, panicky animals, and in cases where a nervous pet chooses it, it can be either used alone or blended with Geranium and Vetiver as a comforting, soothing oil to release tension and trauma. Very good for dominant animals.

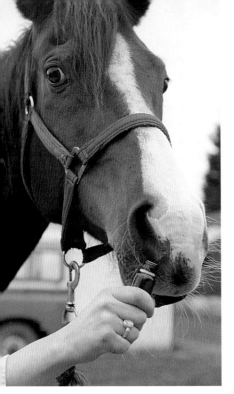

To find out if your horse 'needs' an oil, offer it and watch his reaction. Inhaling deeply through both nostrils indicates interest; indifference or turning away means 'no thanks'.

Citronella oil is the centuries old, fool-proof insect repellent and stimulant, which surprisingly is missed by many practitioners of natural therapies. It is also useful by inhalation for animals with lung conditions. Ideal if diluted in an emulsion of water as a spray insect repellent, but beware of applying to pink skin that may burn in sunlight

Peppermint oil is useful by inhalation as a reviving stimulant during convalescence, for lung conditions, on inflamed injuries such as muscles and joints (but not involving broken skin), and is also a digestive. Occasionally for use (diluted) on the feed of pets with digestive problems or to tempt fussy feeders during times of worry.

Vetiver is, in my experience, the most sedative oil available. It has the effect of drawing in scattered energy and anchoring or grounding it, so is vital in cases of stress, nerves, aggression, tension, anxiety, excitement, trauma, after accident or injury, and so on. Do not use with animals that are depressed as it will exacerbate the condition.

Carrot Seed is the oil I choose for the skin where all else has failed. It is useful in external application (diluted in carrier oil) for healing skin and can be beneficial in cases of scarring, for hair regrowth, and wounds and skin conditions of all kinds. It can be given internally (again diluted) for urinary disorders.

Geranium is balancing, soothing, calming, refreshing and wonderful for the release of tension. A very strong hormonal balancer which is often used together with with Clary sage.

Marigold is another great oil for skin application in all kinds of conditions and is refreshing, uplifting and comforting.

Neroli or **Jasmine** are ideal for stressed, depressed or tense animals.

Garlic is a great insect repellent and for inhalation in lung conditions, as well as a stimulant to the immune system.

SIMPLE OIL BLEND IDEAS

The blends given here are tried-and-tested remedies for animals.

- To repel insects: Citronella, Lavender, Garlic.
- To soothe nerves: Vetiver, Lavender, Neroli.
- To massage inflamed or damaged areas: Peppermint, Carrot Seed, Marigold
- To stimulate: Peppermint, Geranium, Rosemary.
- For skin: Lavender, Marigold, Yarrow.
- For aggression: Clary Sage, Geranium, Jasmine.
- For lungs: Peppermint, Garlic, Eucalyptus or Pine.
- Digestive: Peppermint, Fennel, Carrot Seed.
- While giving energy therapy: Lavender, Jasmine, Geranium or Helichrysum (Immortelle).
- For wounds: Lavender, Tea-tree (but never for dogs).
- For scars: Lavender, Marigold, Camomile.
- For depression: Geranium, Marigold, Jasmine.

PRACTICALITIES OF USING NATURAL REMEDIES

To begin with, use your pet's symptoms as a key to deciding what remedies to use. Once you have decided, see what your pet feels and let him have the final decision. Different therapies can complement and be used alongside each other; for example a soothing and calming oil, a sedative herb, a grounding crystal and a Bach remedy for tension. However, as stressed earlier, do not use everything at once or you will have no clear way of determining the positive or negative effects of the individual remedies. If you do use several remedies in conjunction, make sure that they enhance each other's effects, and not negate them – for example, a stimulating oil might counteract a sedative herb. Many plants can be used in various forms, so once you have made your decision about which plant to go for, experiment with it fresh, dried, as an oil and so on. If you are in any doubt about which remedy to choose or how to use it, consult a detailed text or a practitioner in that field of therapy.

Because energy medicines work to heal the individual on every level, they can have a profound and deep effect. They can provide the way in to problems that exist on a much deeper level and unfold the causes behind physical problems. In the next chapter, I will explain something of the deeper nature of how healing works to move the individual out of a state of dis-ease toward healing.

TOUCHING THE SOUL

So far, I have talked about healing for your animal's physical problems, healing for behavioural issues and the mind/body inter-relationship. By now you will be familiar with the concept of body as manifestation of mind, and the unhappy or stressed mind as the cause behind physical problems.

THE STRESS-FACTOR

What causes the mind to become stressed? Most people would say that animals become stressed as a result of their environment or, more specifically, through discomfort of some kind caused by factors within their environment. This can apply to many levels of the animal's physical existence, from not getting enough food, or the wrong kind of food, not having enough exercise or company, not having the right kind of housing, to being treated aggressively or ignored.

Ultimately, the stress-factor is due to the mind being aware that something isn't right; cues and environmental feedback from the body tell the mind that actually, this is uncomfortable; it's not the situation it wants to be in. For example, hunger causes discomfort, which the mind is well aware of, just as the need to have company or exercise causes discomfort if ignored. The instinctive reaction of the mind is to cause behaviour in the body that seeks to address the discomfort – to find food if the signals are those of hunger, or to move around if the body needs exercise. This kind of discomfort for the mind can therefore be seen as attributable to the animal not doing what it needs or wants to do, and this is the kind of mental stress which can eventually result in physical sickness through suppressed immunity.

The factors influencing an animal's way of life (and thus, stress levels and physical wellbeing) on a day-to-day basis are largely under the control of the person or people who care for that animal. It might seem a bit of an over-statement to say that animals can get sick by not doing or having what they need to do or have. However, if you think about this in terms of getting enough food, it is easy to see that it's not only possible, but also highly likely. Many species of animal have their own specific kinds of behaviour that are a part of their intrinsic nature. For example, cats need to range and go hunting, hamsters need to be active at night and many kinds of dogs need to dig and run as part of their natural behaviour. All of these species-specific behaviours are related to the way that the animal has evolved to survive. The activities that we see our pets engaged in are usually an adapted form of natural, instinctive behaviour related to finding, hunting and gathering food, grooming, mating, maintaining territory and social interaction.

To illustrate, many cats living in cities cannot range or hunt because of busy roads, so their needs have to be curbed, which is not conducive to health. This is why playing 'games' with your cat is a great idea, as it will simulate the chasing and catching activities he would normally enjoy. The innate drives or desires of a dog such as a Border Collie, will include lots of running, which is an adaptive form of chasing or hunting for food. A Border Collie, deprived of the running it needs to do, is likely to become stressed and develop related behavioural problems or physical conditions – which is why it's a good idea to take them for plenty of long walks. Dogs like these are not ideal pets unless you can give them plenty of exercise and attention.

In energetic terms, the basic essence or energy of the cat is directed towards hunting, and the Collie's is directed towards running – it needs to run and can't. So the animal is not doing what it needs to do. The mind of the cat or Collie is simply an interface between its essential needs and its physical existence, and because the two are out of line with each other, the mind is subject to the friction resulting from the rub between what the animal needs and its reality. Voilà! One stressed pet! It is up to each of us who keeps an animal as a companion to provide what that animal most needs, in order to stay happy and, thus, healthy. This can prove tricky for those who live in towns and cities and who still wish to keep pets, and this is why it is so important for all of us to understand the commitment we make to an animal in taking it on. Cats, for instance, provided they get used to it from an early age, adapt very well to an indoor life. But the amount of attention which you'll need to give an animal living in such conditions may be greater than if the cat had the freedom of the garden and the possibility to hunt and climb trees. I always say that people should have an animal as practice for parenthood, because the demands your pet places on your time and imagination can almost equal those of children!

Opposite page: Cats who live in the country often display quasi wild behaviour, going off on long hunting expeditions and roaming over a large territory.

Our pets have deep, innate needs that have to be expressed, not suppressed. This exuberant dog is in his element.

THE SOUL AGENDA

In human terms, the essence or basic driving energy of the individual is often called the soul. Human sickness can therefore also be understood as a result of the friction between what the soul wants or needs, and the physical reality of the individual. People living the kind of life where they aren't able to do what they need to do are usually those who become, initially, stressed or depressed, which in turn leads to illness. They will often ask questions like, 'What's it all about?', 'What's the point of life?' or 'Why am I living like this?' Animals experience comparable depressed feelings but clearly aren't in a position to articulate them to their owners, and it is this kind of depression that can lead to illness for our pets.

The soul or basic essential energy of any individual of any species has its needs, or its own agenda. This is expressed in human terms as having a 'purpose' and it is this purpose that people are trying to get in touch with when they ask what life means, or what the 'point' is. For humans this can be quite a complex

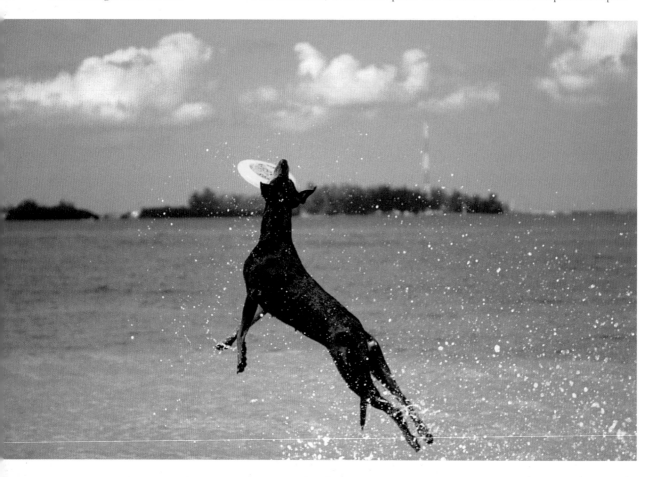

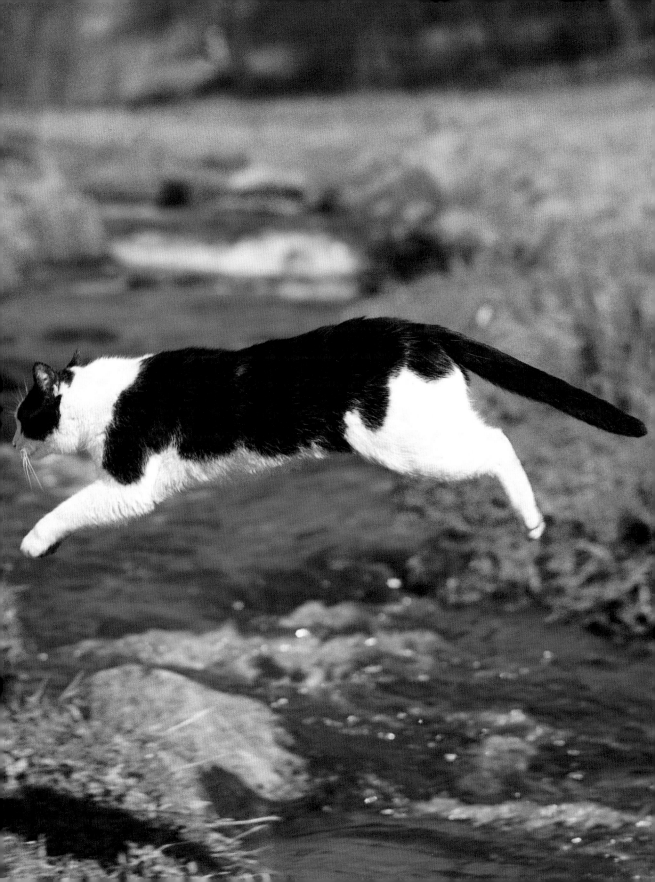

process; their 'purpose' or 'need' is often related to the strengths or talents that each individual has. Often, these strengths or talents are learned through experiences in life, and not just something that the individual is born with. One individual might have especially loving energies and a need to direct these to caring for other people. It might be said of such a person that his or her 'soul agenda' is caring for others. If this individual worked as a nurse, his or her life would be a pretty happy, fulfilled, satisfying place to be – using his or her energies to help others in the best way possible. If a totally different profession is chosen, the rub or friction between the individual's energies or soul agenda and the reality of how that individual spends the bulk of his or her working life, could cause a deal of stress that might be difficult to live with.

For people, knowing the soul agenda isn't always easy. It is said that, as the energetic essence of the soul enters the unborn body, the form of that energy has total awareness – it knows exactly what it needs to do, what energies are strongest, and which are weakest, so will be enhanced by joining with or seeking other energies. The purpose, or energetic needs of the essence is to seek other energetic input to enhance or balance itself. New energetic input is found, learned or developed through experience. In this way, it can be said that life is about healing the soul; balancing the essential energies of the individual at the most basic level. I believe that we come into life with a purpose or agenda and fulfil that in order to balance or heal our energy, through directing our strongest energies where they will benefit others and through seeking balancing or developing influences to our energies.

Often if you ask a child what they want to 'be', they will know quite clearly what their purpose is, or what kind of energies they have, how these could best be directed or simply what it would make them most happy to do. They don't have the 'clutter' that we do as adults. Some people hold that vision through to adulthood, or come to know what their need or purpose is through being aware and knowing their own nature very well. For other adults, who have been conditioned to perceive certain activities as more worthy than others, and to see factors such as money or material possessions as more important than simple 'happiness', the soul agenda can get lost, forgotten or simply ignored. The least healthy people are often the ones who are living in physical situations that, when it comes down to it, they just don't want to be in. Their sickness is a result of their discomfort and often provides an excuse for them not to have to go in to uncomfortable situations (for example, being sick can be a great way to avoid a meeting at work, or a maths lesson at school). So the way to heal them is to help them to find out what they truly need or want, and to encourage them to make the necessary changes to their life.

Before we can attempt to heal a problem, we need first to know how to get in touch with the energetic essence to discover the individual agenda – we need to learn how to touch the soul.

ANIMALS – OUR SOULMATES

The soul agenda of most animals is nowhere near as complex as that of humans because they don't have the kind of complicated existence or the issues that we do. The essential energies, or soul agenda, of many animals that man is attracted to as a companion are strongest on the frequencies that elicit feelings of companionship, warmth, calm, comfort and love from humans. This is primarily because many of the animals we choose as our companions are pack or group animals, so their energies are concerned with bonding to companions. You could almost say that many animals are born with part of their soul agenda as giving unconditional love to their human companions – their energies are balanced by being in the situation where they give and receive companionship. Conversely, humans experience life as quite an individual experience and seek the security of companionship. The needs of humans and animals thus provide a basis for a balanced relationship.

To heal our animals, then, we need to understand their individual soul agenda and how we can fulfil that in physicality. I should say at this point that in my experience this is really only an issue for animals like cats, dogs and larger animals. I have worked with many animals that were just plain 'unhappy' with their lives, which resulted in depression, stress and sickness. Sometimes this is clear to an outsider, but not so clear if you're in the situation and, particularly, if you have an agenda of your own that adds to the animal's problems. For example, I have treated cats that were used for showing and led quite unnatural lives, that would much rather have been out and about enjoying themselves. A change in their lifestyle, allowing them more access to the great outdoors, improved their health and outlook beyond measure. I once worked on a gun dog, who spent his life in a pen outside, and was only given human attention and affection on shooting days or when he was exercised. He was a particularly

'You could almost say that many animals are born with part of their soul agenda as giving unconditional love to their human companions – their energies are balanced by being in the situation where they give and receive companionship.'

sad little dog, who wanted nothing more than to have some companionship in his life – a problem that was easily solved by a little more thought on his owner's part, and a new playmate to share his pen. Horses, more often than any other animals, have their needs ignored in favour of what is convenient and suitable to the owner. One horse I treated simply hated being ridden, and though he was very difficult to manage, his owner's agenda was that she ride him. She failed to see what he was showing her until it got to the point where his behaviour made him impossible to ride. He is much happier and healthier just being a horse in a field with some companions. As with people, once the soul agenda can be brought into line with physical life, the friction created by unfulfilled needs simply disappears and physical and mental wellbeing follow. One way to get in touch with the soul is to use energy as a means of communication.

CONTACT

Contact is defined as: 'a condition or state of touching, meeting or communicating; electrical connection for the passage of current.' It's a word that plays a big part in healing the soul.

Some people develop such a close relationship and deep understanding with their pets that they feel that they can really communicate with each other, just by a look or a touch.

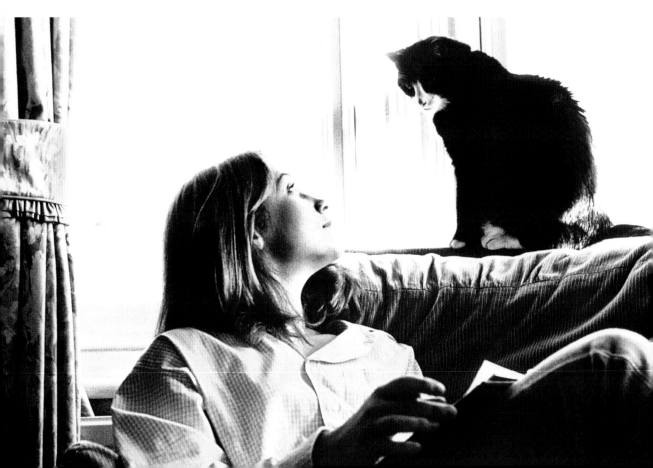

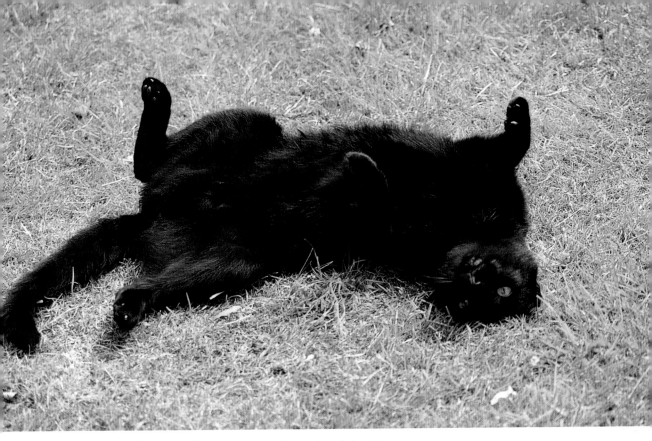

In Chapter 3, under the heading 'Assessing energy', I mentioned that it is not uncommon to receive impressions or thoughts as a result of the energetic exchange between individuals. The way your brain interprets the thoughts, as pictures or words (and sometimes even smells and sounds) is simply its way of processing the energetic impulses it receives. This kind of information exchange through energy is called all kinds of things, such as clairvoyance, E.S.P., telepathy, psychic ability or, with animals, 'animal communication'. The idea of an 'energetic information internet' has also been called 'the collective conscious' by the psychologist Jung. It's seen as a way for individuals to pick up on each others' energetic impulses, sharing of the energetic element that we can all tune into.

Experts in energy now understand that the world as an energetic field means that perception of information within that field is, quite simply, a reality. People and animals can pick up all kinds of different energetic impulses from each other, such as thoughts, feelings, imprints of experiences and so on (how else do the animal-heroes I mentioned in Chapter 5 know what the humans they save need?).

Many people who begin to work with energy to heal report an increase in sensitivity to energies of all kinds. The best way to increase your own sensitivity or raise your awareness to energetic frequencies is simply to practise healing as much as possible, or to take some kind of healing-energy attunement (as I described in Chapter 2, under the heading 'Getting started'). Energy has all kinds of different frequencies and those that we 'tune into' for healing match many of the vibrations within the body, mind and soul of the individuals we work with using energy, be they animal or human. The exchange of impressions, ideas or information during treatments can develop your own awareness of the energies you are working with, and in this way you can learn, with experience, to 'tune into' or listen to your animals' essential energy, or soul.

For example, once when I was working on a man who had asked to feel what healing energy was like, I just put my hands on him and instantly received the impression of him sitting in a worn armchair in the evening, smoking a cigarette and watching television. The feeling was of him being tired out at the end of a hard day. So, it was quite natural for me to say to him, 'You know, you need to slow down a little – and cut out the smoking. You're not giving yourself enough time to relax in the evening'. This was simply my brain's way of interpreting the impulses it received from the man, and translating it into a response. As it was, he agreed, but was surprised that I should be able to tell all of this from a simple touch.

Exactly the same kind of exchange can take place with animals. I once put my hands on a dog and had an impression of him feeling really insecure and low-down in the pecking order, because his owner also has three other dogs. He constantly fought with the others because he wanted to be closer to the head of the pack – his owner. I had no idea whether there were other dogs in the house at the time, but his owner confirmed my impressions. My response was to suggest that this dog be given special 'time out', even for as little as ten minutes each day, but to be with his owner without the competition for attention from the other dogs. I suppose the most dramatic case of seeing what a horse felt was an occasion where it was clear to me that the little old chap, tired and sick, just wanted to die, but was 'hanging on' for his owners' sake (more of this in Chapter 8). Of course, the impressions I gain are simply my brain's way of translating the energetic impulses it receives. Some people call this 'talking to' animals, but it's simply the exchange of energy and is something everyone can learn to do given time, practice, patience and sensitivity.

THE HEALER WITHIN

The person or practitioner giving the treatment, then, is certainly not the 'healer'. All that individual does is act a little like a telephone wire: connecting the soul of the being you are working on with the energetic source from which it came. I explain this process to pupils of mine as a little like the process where E.T. phones home! The creature, feeling isolated, hurt, unhappy or confused, needs to find some way of gaining comfort; of re-establishing itself and its own energy, which in turn facilitates the healing process. The healing process itself is therefore one involving the practitioner as the catalyst or connection (rather like a jump-lead); the link or contact between energies. Some therapists describe this process as getting in touch with the 'well' part of the individual (some call it the 'health'), the place where the soul is at ease and knows what it needs to do. Buddhists call this wellness or propensity for re-establishing balance and harmony the 'Buddha nature' within.

In effect, the 'phoning home', or contact with source energy, gives the soul being healed access to fresh energy and strength, which can result in an energetic shift, enabling healing on every level, including the physical body. Some people call this the process of realization or enlightenment – of bringing in the light, or energy, to the struggling soul energy of the individual. The healer, therefore, is within each and every living being – in the divine spark of pure energy which, when contacted, enables the soul agenda to realign with the physical existence.

> *'The way to improve your own clarity is to work as much with energy as possible and to allow yourself to become clear in mind and body.'*

THE PRACTITIONER'S ROLE

By touching the soul, we make ourselves available as the contact between forms of energy. By listening to the soul, we can help to identify and interpret the soul agenda and help to bring this into reality. All we're really doing is hand-holding on a soul level and the most important element of this is simply to make ourselves available as a mechanism by which this can be allowed to happen. It's almost like the old adage of 'tea and sympathy'; all we need to do is simply be there; listen, acknowledge the animal's suffering and recognize that this individual is seeking healing. This recognition and reconnection with the larger energy source can release the energetic tension causing illness and allow the soul to come through and experience wellbeing. This is why I tell people that in learning to heal, they are simply choosing to become a 'tool'.

The healing that takes place through connection of the soul energy to its source can be likened to counselling on an energetic level – the energetic release of the individual's trauma and negativity by providing a safe and unconditional environment in which that can happen. Often, this powerful process takes place as the culmination of sickness, pain or confusion having led to this moment. Connection provides the opportunity to find a way forward, to move the energy. The events leading to this situation have actually formed part of the individual's life journey or learning experience, part of the development, balancing and thus, healing of the energetic essence of that individual.

As the practitioner is simply a connection, it follows that people involved in this kind of work need to be (and often naturally are) a clear route (some people call this a 'channel') for energy of all kinds. This happens of its own accord as people start to work with energy, which always helps to heal the person working with it, too, even while giving a treatment to another person or animal. The way to improve your own clarity is to work as much with energy as possible and to allow yourself to become clear in mind and body. Some people take up meditation or some other form of spiritual development practice in order to find a clear place in their own minds. Meditation is really a big word for doing nothing – it's all about silencing your mental chatter and being at peace. Some people change their diets or give up smoking or alcohol to help de-stress and detoxify their physical and energetic bodies. Any energies coming through you will be less strong if they're getting stuck on the way, because you're giving them lots of extra work to do on your own body.

All we actually do in healing practice is learn to tune in to certain frequencies of energy. As you become more sensitive, you can learn to distinguish different frequencies of energy and listen to your animals. Many of you are already doing this, and just need practice to learn how to tune your attention or focus to each frequency of energy. For most people, this doesn't come overnight, but evolves as a steady process of receiving impressions during healing treatments and making sense of them. Gradually, as you begin to receive these kinds of impressions, you learn to 'look for' or tune into that place or frequency of energy within the individual, to allow impressions to come through.

It is important to remain calm, focused and non-judgmental. Many people who spend lots of time with animals have a habit of interpreting their animals' looks, expressions and behaviour – e.g. 'He says he wants his dinner now!'

Opposite page. In this picture I'm about to treat Mole, my Arab stallion. Before I begin, I always 'ask permission', to check that he really wants a treatment. This shot captures the moment of my question and his acceptance.

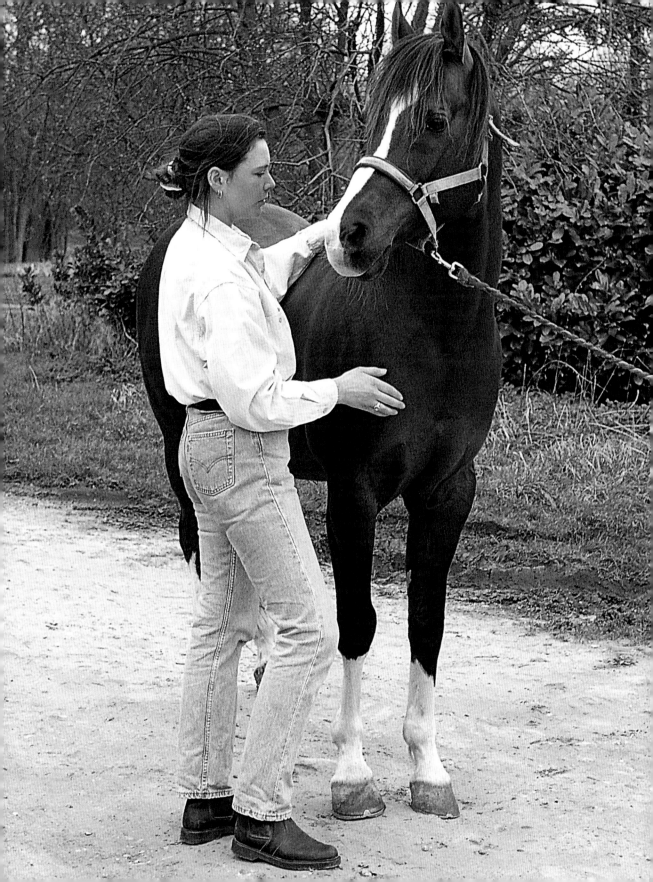

Whilst much of this is valid and does involve genuine perception of what an animal is attempting to communicate, beware that you are not projecting your own thoughts and feelings onto your animals – 'She will be very annoyed if you call her fat!' People habitually do this as a way to express their own feelings – it's known as 'projection' in psychology. However, this isn't very helpful in a healing situation.

The way to learn to distinguish between your own thoughts and input from the animal is simply to still your own mental noise and to remain open to impressions that come unbidden into your conscious. You will become sharply aware of impressions from outside (the first reaction is to think, 'where did that come from?'); and thoughts or ideas of your own. In reality they feel totally different and you quickly learn to distinguish what comes from the animal you are working on, because you would never have thought of it for yourself. It's all about leaving your own 'stuff' out of the way and just letting things happen. If you find yourself unable to work in this way without introducing your own ideas, it's as well to take up some form of mental practice (like meditation) to learn to put your own thoughts to one side. There is also a question of confidence involved. People often fail to trust impressions they receive intuitively because they worry about their validity. Patience and practice are the most valuable teachers.

If you are working to help heal someone else's animal, you also need to learn to act as the go-between for the animal and the humans around it, who may be quite out of touch with the animal's needs. In this case you are entirely responsible for what you pass on to the people in that situation about impressions you have received from the animal. This is a situation which requires tact and empathy with the feelings of the people and animals involved. It is as well to pass on only what is necessary for the animal's healing, and not to add your own thoughts, opinions or advice, unless expressly asked. Remember, you are simply offering healing and may not be an expert in animal behaviour! If in doubt, be honest and simply say: 'I don't know'. You start out by listening and, if necessary, interpreting. Then if people need some input in practical terms you can add it to help them find a way forward.

Most people are happy and willing to do whatever they need to do to help their animals to recover from illness or unhappiness. Sometimes, though, it isn't easy for people to accept that they need to make radical changes to help their animal to get well, particularly if, like our show cat, gun dog or riding horse, the animal would rather have a different role in life. Sometimes, people want you to get in there and tell their animals to jolly well sort themselves out, which is the owner's agenda, and not that of the animal involved. Cases like these can prove problematic until the owner accepts what the animal really wants or needs. It may take some time for the person to understand or absorb the facts and much tact in the presentation of the information on your part. You should always, at some point, check if what you are doing is OK with the animal you are working with. This is a vital point and one that I cannot stress too highly. Remember, the animal will only heal as and when it is ready to do so. Occasionally, an animal will withdraw from this kind of close healing contact; often, when it's very sick, it simply wants to be left alone. It can be very difficult to have to tell someone that a much-loved animal has had enough of its life, and just wants to be released.

OLD AGE AND LETTING GO

Most of us choose to have animals as our companions because we love having their company. We become very attached to them and number our animals among our closest friends and companions. Those who have animals as opposed to children often think of their pets as their children. For me, animals are my constant companions, friends, guides and teachers. They give comfort in difficult times, share all the fun (they create a lot of it), are involved in my most magical experiences and, of course, are an endless source of unconditional love in a way that few humans are. Many of us, myself included (due to the nature of my work), spend more time in the company of animals than with people.

GETTING OLD AND SLOWING DOWN

The hardest part of sharing your life with any animal is that we live so much longer than most of our pets do. Consequently, we often witness the process of natural ageing and death in our pets. Some animals, will live to a completely healthy old age, with relatively few problems, and simply die quietly at home. Many animals, though, however well cared for, begin to suffer from various health problems as they age, purely through wear and tear and the natural process of ageing.

Many species of animal will experience the ageing process as a need to slow down. As the body becomes less capable of sustaining the same levels of activity that it did in earlier life, animals need a little extra care and attention and a little less activity. As the body ages, some of the functions that it performs start to flag or operate less efficiently. This might mean that your pet puts on weight or loses weight, or needs a special diet that is adapted to suit a less tolerant digestive system. He may play less and want less exercise, or prefer gentle exercise in small doses instead. His hearing or eyesight may deteriorate, and he may become less mobile than he formerly was.

Just because the health problems that your pet suffers are related to old age, this is no excuse not to give him healing treatments on a regular basis. I recently heard one man say of his cat, 'Well, he's sixteen. What can you expect?' You can

Opposite. Our pets can become our closest companions and our relationship with them may even outlast human ones. There is real truth at times in the concept of man's *best* friend!

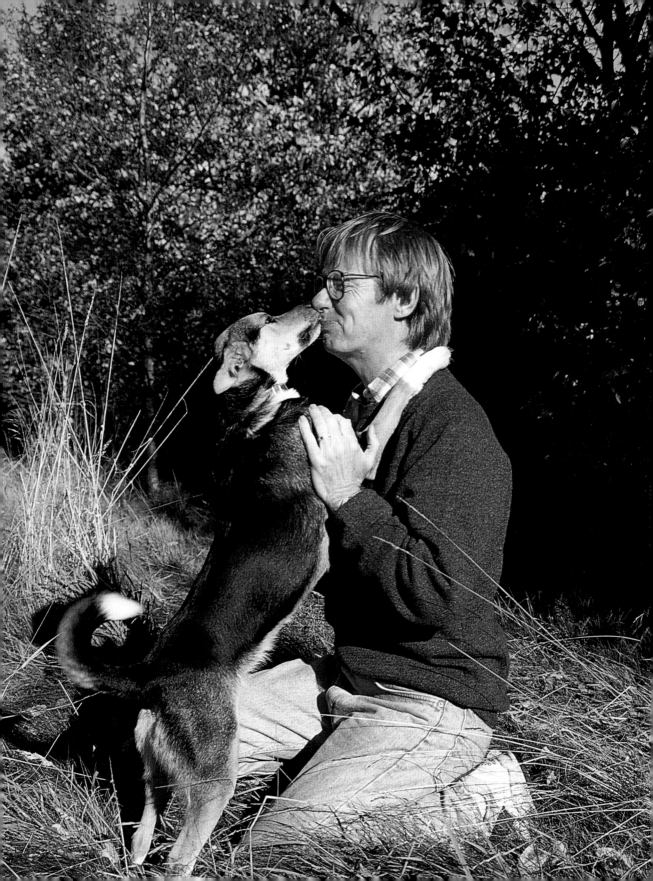

expect to give your pet a comfortable old age, not to write him off because he's getting on in years. Giving treatments to your pet helps to ensure that his energy levels are constantly topped up and that he remains well and does not fall prey to disease or weakness. Treatments can also help to ease the discomfort of many of the conditions that older pets suffer, such as degeneration of the joints.

If your pet has a particular health problem, you can also combat it using other vibrational medicines. Herbal preparations such as Devils' Claw and Cider Vinegar can work wonders for mobility, while other remedies such as Slippery Elm and Meadowsweet are good for maintaining a healthy digestive system. You can combine healing treatments with some gentle massage using small, steady circular movements all over your pet's body. Dogs in particular will appreciate the addition of a relaxing essential oil such as Lavender as part of the treatment – cats are generally happier being massaged without any oil. Sessions like this can help to free up stiff muscles, maintain circulation and enhance mobility in stiff joints. If he will let you, softly massaging the gums and lips (without oil), as well as the paws and ears, is a deeply therapeutic treatment and can help your dog or cat to let go of physical tension and encourage quiet, peaceful sleep. These gentle but enjoyable 'massages' can help to make life easier for ageing animals.

HEALING ISN'T ALWAYS CURING

Sometimes, when you treat animals with healing energy therapy, they make a remarkable recovery – even when they're supposedly 'terminally' ill. Sometimes, they get better surely but steadily. Sometimes, they don't improve. People can find it hard to understand how one animal can die whilst another has recovered. It's all about timing and what the animal is ready to do and capable of doing. This comes back down to the animal's individual agenda – not that of the humans around him. So, sometimes, healing isn't curing. Sometimes, healing means helping the animal to die in a relaxed, peaceful and comfortable way. Sometimes, it just means helping your pet to die less painfully.

Not being 'cured' is the option of the individual. If you think about the soul as the vital energetic essence of an animal, you will obviously have ideas about where that energy came from before it was embodied in the animal's physical existence, and what happens to it after the animal's body dies. In nature, things don't simply start or stop existing – they merely change. Nature is rounded and cyclic – so the food I eat helps to form my body, which when it dies, will go back into the ground to provide food for another form of life – insects, plants and so on. It's the same with energy; it doesn't cease to be, it simply changes form.

QUALITY OF LIFE

When pets reach old age and their health begins to fail, many owners suffer agonies over their pets' quality of life. Is he happy? Is he in pain? Does he mind being in pain, so long as he can still do what he wants to do? Can he move OK? Should we keep him going on drugs? Would he be happier if I just let him go? These are big questions for owners and generally quite difficult to be objective about. It's hard to assess your pet's quality of life without clouding his experiences with your own emotions. This is where working with energy can provide a valuable way for us to listen to what our pets really want and need.

Sometimes, when I am asked to work on an animal, I put my hands on him and find that the animal is very withdrawn and has quite a low energy. This is typical of an animal who is winding down because he has had enough – enough treatments, enough messing about, and enough life. When you do get into an interaction on an energetic level, it becomes apparent that actually, he is ready to die. He just wants to be let go. If you treat your pet with an open and sensitive mind, as I explained in the previous chapter, he will let you know quite clearly when he no longer wants to live. You won't be in any doubt.

The owners or 'family' of an animal who has had enough, however, can find this really hard to accept and just want the animal to get better somehow and live longer. Although, in fact, this is quite a selfish view, it's understandable given how attached we become to our pets. What happens in situations like these is that the animal gets the energetic signals from the owners – 'Don't go! Stay with us!' Hanging on can cause problems for the animal that wants to go but feels held. Animals subjected to such pressure will often struggle to keep going until their health fails them completely, or until the people around them finally realize that enough is enough, and give the animal permission to die. Once this happens, most animals are so relieved that they let go quite quickly of their own accord.

A friend of mine tells a story about his old cat, Fang, who had been with him since he was a tiny kitten. Fang was getting on in years and one day was clearly exhausted, ill, and very depressed. My friend remembers watching Fang for a day or two, and realizing that his cat has simply 'had enough', but seemed to be

Opposite page. Living with an ageing animal can be deeply rewarding. An old dog or cat may not play as boisterously as he once did but he'll repay his owner with unfailing devotion and a new gentleness. Healing energy therapy can help keep your pet healthy and happy through his old age and ease his final moments when the time comes.

An older animal will benefit from the addition of parsley to its food. This herb relieves aches and pains, stimulates blood circulation and the heart, keeps the urinary tracts working properly.

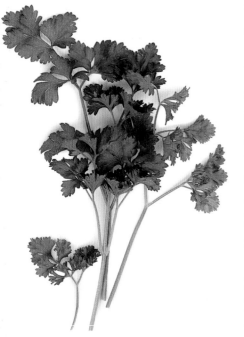

awaiting permission to go. He held Fang in his arms and said to him, 'It's OK, friend, don't you worry, you go now', and Fang let go there and then, literally dying in his owners' arms. My friend says he felt a real sense of relief from his cat as he spoke the words that seemed to release his hold on his little companion.

Some pets are lucky enough to die naturally. Others, however, have to be put to sleep because their health has degenerated so much that they really have had enough and want to be let go. Sometimes, animals suffer from sudden accidents and are in such deep pain that they would rather be helped to die, rather than suffering a '50/50' operation or prolonged trauma. I remember working on one horse that was clearly in terrible pain from an accidental blow to his leg, but his vet felt that there was a chance he could pull through, given time. The horse simply couldn't bear the pain – every time he tried to move, his heart jumped as he almost 'winced' outwardly. He had shut off completely from the people and other horses around him, and simply wanted to die. Having attempted to keep him going for a week or so, his owner recognized her horse's suffering and knew it would be far kinder to put him to sleep than to keep him hanging on in such pain. The decision to have your pet put down needn't be agonizing, however, if you just listen to him and allow him to tell you how he would be happiest. If you really can't hear, sometimes he'll just make it obvious by appearing to give up the will to live, as the horse I mentioned did – he stopped eating, his coat began to fall out, and he just stood still.

Being put to sleep can come as a blessed relief for an animal who is suffering but feels that he is not allowed to die. It's not a mean thing to do – sometimes it's the most compassionate thing. I have heard several of my human clients, often people in hospital who have suffered a long or painful illness, say that they just wish it could all be over – that they have had enough and would really like to go. They say their goodbyes, and slip away quite naturally. With the best of intentions, people are sometimes kept alive by medical intervention when all quality of life, and will to live, has gone. Human euthanasia is illegal, no matter how cruel the sustenance of life may seem at times. However, we can do this final service for our animals when they reach this condition.

LETTING GO, AND SAYING GOODBYE

Being with your pet as he dies naturally is a great privilege and can help to ease the pain of loss. Animals often choose to die alone, in a comfortable place where

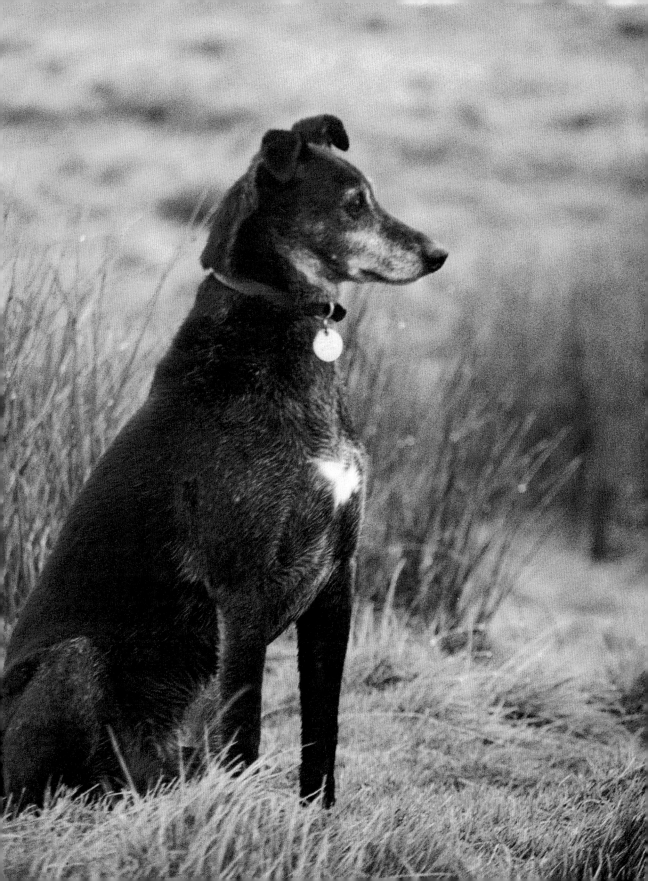

they feel safe. Occasionally, owners are quite relieved to be spared the experience; on the other hand, others prefer to be involved so that they can let go and say goodbye. Someone whose pet has died in an accident when they weren't around can feel a greater sense of loss because they missed the opportunity to share their pet's last moments. One positive aspect for owners who do have to make the decision of having their pets put to sleep is that they can make a choice about whether to be involved or not at the time of death.

Being with your pet as he lets go of his physical body and his energy is released into a new form of existence is a profoundly moving experience and one that many pet owners are glad to have been part of. If you treat your pet softly with energy as he is dying, you will not only make his passage more peaceful, gentle and comfortable, but you will also be helping to heal your pet's energy as it moves into a new form. Animals who are given healing at the time of death often close their eyes, sigh and let go without a struggle. Holding your pet or laying a hand on him as he dies, can ensure that his last moments are peaceful, pleasant and relaxed and that you are there to support him during the transition of energy from the physical body.

SAYING THANK YOU

If you are involved in your pet's death, whether he dies naturally at home or is put to sleep at the vet's surgery, it is important to make him feel completely loved and at peace as he dies. Sadly this is the moment that so many of us struggle with and we end up sobbing uncontrollably, so the last experience we have with that soul is a sad one. I feel that we should make every effort possible to let go with thanks and love, and to send our pets forward with our sincerest wishes for the best possible existence in whatever form. Actually this is a fairly Buddhist viewpoint. In Buddhism, it is believed that the point of death should be graceful, supported and surrounded by peaceful good wishes for the dying soul. It is beneficial to a dying animal if we can remain calm and give thanks and good wishes as he leaves his body. The animal dies with a feeling of relief and deep peace, as opposed to one of guilt and trauma for leaving his human companions behind.

If you know that your pet is dying or are taking him to be put to sleep, it can be a wonderful last memory to share a final special occasion together before he dies. Whatever your pet most enjoys doing or whatever your were happiest doing together is obviously the best choice, as long as it is physically possible for your pet. It might be a last gentle game together, or a little walk, or sitting in a special place, or simply a peaceful cuddle. Whatever you do, it should take on the form of a celebration of thanks for the time you have shared with your pet.

In practical terms, your pet should be made as comfortable as possible as he dies. It can be a comfort to your pet to take him to his favourite place if he is unable to move of his own accord. You can place him in his own bed, surround him with familiar and comfortable objects and lay your hand on his body to give energy as he passes away. One client of mine took her cat's beanbag and placed it on her own pillow as she felt the time was drawing near for her cat to let go and die. She placed her cat on the beanbag next to her head and fell asleep stroking her; when she woke up later during the night, her cat seemed to have passed away quietly as they both slept. It can be a good idea to keep other animals and children away unless you are certain that they won't disturb the dying animal. Remember to thank him and let him know that your love goes with him.

CELEBRATING LIFE

Whether your pet is buried at home, cremated, or buried at a special pet's cemetery, marking his passing with a funeral ceremony offers a way of acknowledging the joy that he brought into your life, and of saying goodbye. You can make as much or as little of this as you choose and, especially when there are children in the family, this last goodbye provides a way of saying thank you in a very individual way for all the joy your pet has brought to the family. The animal can be buried in his favourite blanket or with his favourite toy, with a photograph, flower or poem. My friend made a beautiful wooden casket for Fang to be buried in, and he let his little cat lie 'in state' for a couple of days so that all the family could say their goodbyes, before burying the casket in the garden. Your ceremony could include playing music, and family members can share memories of your pet, or perhaps read a special poem. Whatever you do, a funeral should be a celebration – a marking of the passage of a special and wonderful creature.

If your pet is cremated, you can opt to have the ashes returned to you to keep, or scatter in a favourite spot. Or, you can have him buried or his ashes kept at a special pet cemetery, so that you can visit his grave. You might feel that it is an important part of your grieving process to be able to visit a grave and tend it, a

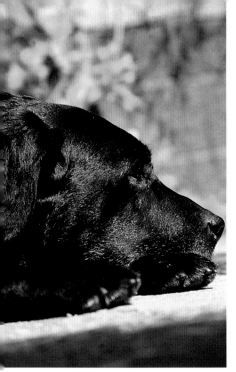

Just as we mourn the loss of our pets, they miss a companion who dies. If you have an animal whose playmate has died, give energy to the remaining pet, who may feel lost and sad.

way of cherishing the memory of your pet's life; somewhere you can go to think about the special times you shared together. One of the most memorable ways to mark a pet's grave at home is with a specially chosen natural stone or by planting a shrub to mark the place. Rosemary is a good choice as it signifies remembrance.

COPING WITH LOSS

For most of us, the period following the death of a much-loved pet can be a difficult time of adjustment and grieving. Feelings of loss and grief are entirely natural, particularly if your pet was your main companion, or a big part of your family life. It is important that you allow yourself time to grieve if you need to, in the same way as you would for the loss of a human companion. Buddhists would say that the best way to prepare for death is to live each moment as if it were your last. This has a truth for anyone who has companion animals. Although, of course, we all wish for our animals to live to a ripe old age, it is worth bearing their mortality in mind. Only by being aware of the fragility of life and seeing it as the precious gift that it is, can we appreciate every moment that we spend with our pets. Cherishing your pet and the special gift of time you have together can help you to feel less traumatized by his passing. Rather than regretting the time you didn't spend together, you can remain calm and fulfilled knowing that you really did live every moment you had with each other. Without regrets about letting your animal go, your feeling will be one of gratitude toward the creature who came into your life and a deep appreciation of the time you shared.

The energetic soul of each being comes into a physical existence to balance and develop to the point of wholeness and healing. For most souls, this takes place over the course of many lifetimes, each being a process of learning and development. Sometimes, individuals die because their soul has done what it came to do – learned what it needed to learn this time and is now moving on to another existence. Sometimes, a soul struggles with a particular learning experience and needs to come back in a different existence to learn how to move forwards. Many souls have links with each other between one existence and another and seek to balance their experiences together over more than one lifetime. Sometimes, the animals we share our lives with have been our teachers, companions and friends before, and will be again. Some people are even lucky enough to recognize the soul of an animal they have had the pleasure to know once in this lifetime already, returning in another existence.

Each lifetime is a process of learning, gaining experience and moving forward. We learn a great deal from each of the animals that touch our lives and, though it can be hard to see or understand at the time, each and every situation, no matter how hard, is an opportunity to learn. One of the main ways that I advise people to cope with the grief of losing a much-loved pet is to reflect on what you have learned with your pet during your life together. This can provide a key to moving forward – taking what you have learned and offering it for the benefit of a different animal or individual. In this way, you truly can thank your pet for coming into your life and how he has prepared you for the next stage.

Throughout the grieving process, treat yourself with healing energy as much as you can and as often as feel you need it. It will help to release your emotions, enable you to move forward mentally and to maintain your energy levels and wellbeing. Bach Flower Remedies are ideal for self-administration at such times of change: Rescue Remedy for shock and emotional upheaval; Walnut, to help with the process of change; and Star of Bethlehem, White Chestnut and Oak are all helpful at times of loss. Valerian, Hops and Passionflower can have a calming effect, while infusions of Camomile and Lemon Balm, taken in the evening, can help you to sleep peacefully.

Grieving for the loss of a loved companion takes time, and the process can be so painful or the memories of your pet so strong that you might think you will never have another animal. Often, though, these are the thoughts of a moment of emotional turmoil and most people in time look for a new animal as a companion. In my friend's case, a new kitten found him some time after his cat Fang had died – it simply turned up in his barn one day and stayed. He didn't know if he was ready to take on another cat – but the kitten decided for him, and they became good friends. For other people, the best way to cope with having lost one animal is to give their love and attention to another as soon as possible as a way of healing the past. Either way, a new animal in the household makes for an exciting time, often accompanied by a steep learning curve!

ENERGY FOR A NEW LIFE

When animals are born or a new pet is welcomed into the household, there can follow quite a tumultuous time for all concerned as part of the settling-in and adjustment process. A new relationship of any kind can be fascinating, surprising, confusing, full of ups and downs, but, of course, always incredibly rewarding. New relationships with animals aren't so very different from new relationships with people. It's all about communication – when people don't know each other very well, they can get their wires crossed, and this happens just as frequently (if not more often!) with our animals. The most important point to remember is that it's all about learning to live with each other. It's not about dominating your pet or making rules; it's about finding out how you can best get along and be happy together. It's a learning process on both sides – yours and the animal's.

MAKING BABIES

There's nothing more likely to melt the human heart than the sight of a bundle of tiny, velvet-skinned puppies all dozing gently together or learning to play and tumble on unsteady legs. There's nothing guaranteed to open up the affections of even the hardest, strongest man, than a bunch of new-born kittens with bright blue eyes, fuzzy coats and tiny pink feet. Young animals appeal to the human instincts of caring and protection in a deeply powerful and direct way. Sadly the human mind is somewhat fickle and a lot of the things that those little darlings do, once removed from the safety of their mothers, are more like a test of endurance and tolerance than the ideal picture of a permanently wide-eyed miniature animal that we had envisaged.

People who have female pets often think about breeding from them, partly for fun and partly to have a youngster as a 'chip off the old block'. If you are thinking about breeding from a domestic pet, my advice generally is don't. There are so many unwanted animals in the world. Animal shelters are full to bursting and it makes much more sense, if you're looking for a young animal, to give a home to one that really needs it rather than adding to the problem. A far more responsible approach is to neuter animals of breeding age. However, accidents do happen and sometimes heart rules head, so motherhood is something that some pet owners are involved in helping their animals to cope with.

For some reason, we expect animals to take to motherhood and be perfect examples of nature in all its glory as part of the circle of creating new life. However, there is no reason why every female animal should love motherhood any more than a human mother does. Some animals will have a more comfortable pregnancy than others, have more energy or feel tired, eat well or not feel hungry, or put on lots of weight that can cause related physical discomfort in the joints and back, particularly, as well as muscular pain. Carrying a tummy full of ten puppies in the middle of summer isn't the most fun, either.

Coping with an expectant mother involves providing a caring and supportive environment with as little stress and as healthy an input as possible. You can give healing energy treatments right through pregnancy, which helps the mother in all kinds of ways – not least by stilling the wriggling youngsters inside. Of course, by treating the mother, you are also giving energy to the unborn young, which is an immensely humbling and privileged situation to find yourself in. To offer healing to the life that is still forming is quite something. Usually you find that all movement stills as you work – it's almost as if the young go to sleep, which provides a welcome relief for the mother. It can also bring about quite a feeling of connection between you and the unborn young.

The mother, of course, will appreciate the energetic input on a regular basis and you will find that switched-on animals will keep coming and asking for input quite frequently. Treatments also help to deal with any pain, fatigue or other physical discomfort and to maintain the health of the body, which, in turn, helps to produce healthy young. Some mothers will lose a lot of their own physical resources to a litter, so treating the mother can help to establish a balanced body. Occasionally, expectant mothers can become distressed by the experience (they get that feeling of 'I just want it over with' just like humans do!), and experience difficulties in sleeping, so healing treatments can help to calm and relax them.

A word of warning – take great care with other natural remedies during pregnancy, as many can have adverse effects on the ability of the animal to go to full term, or can affect the unborn young. Essential oils, in particular, should be avoided unless used by an expert. Bach flower remedies are completely safe when used in dilution with spring water, but I wouldn't give them neat because of the alcohol content, which could be unfair on the growing embryo. I recommend Oak, Walnut and Olive during pregnancy. Some herbs are also not advisable for use during pregnancy as they can induce labour, so again, only use a remedy with expert advice.

Make sure that the diet of the expectant mother is well balanced and that adequate gentle exercise is maintained. Dried Raspberry leaves, fed occasionally in small doses (no more than 5g/1–2 teaspoons) can help to strengthen the uterus and discourage haemorrhage during pregnancy. As well as encouraging a healthy labour they can help with cleansing of the afterbirth.

THE MAGICAL MOMENT

The point of birth is an experience like no other. Most animals, though, unless very carefully watched (which can be quite an invasive process), will prefer to birth alone and undisturbed by over-excited human company. Should you

A new life is an incredible gift. The mare puts so much of her own self and nourishment into her foal, ensuring that he grows up robust and healthy.

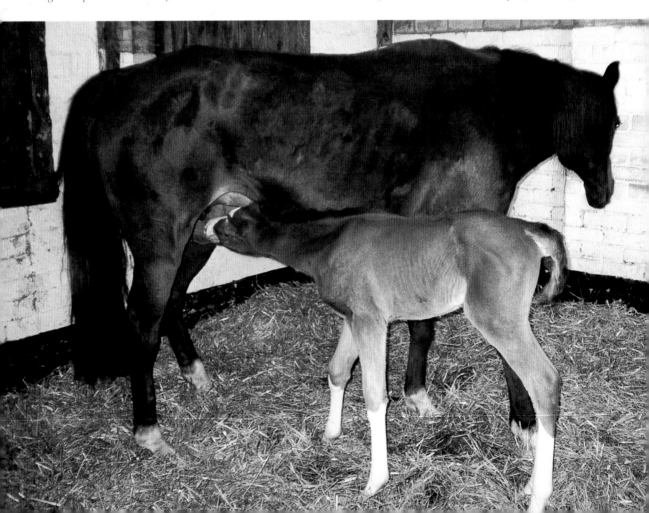

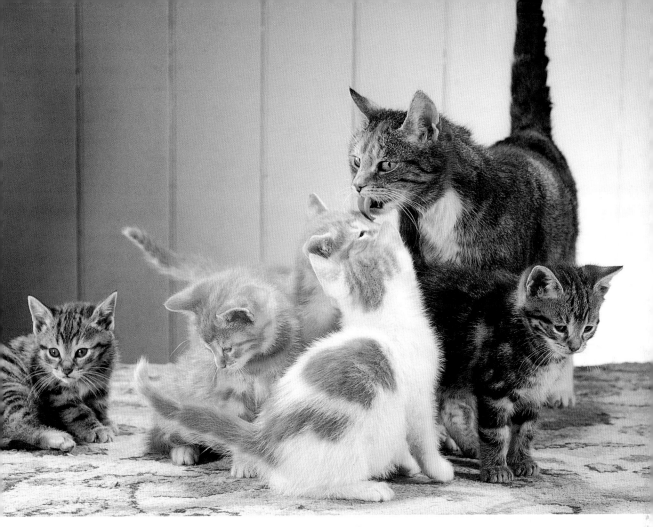

happen to witness the occasion, be prepared for some new and powerful emotions. Bearing witness to the entry into the world of a tiny animal is incredibly moving.

So what can you do, practically, if you are there? Giving healing to the mother during birth helps her to maintain her energy levels, which can make for an easier and less traumatic time during labour. You should do this as gently and quietly as possible, and only if the mother is happy and at ease with what you are doing. You can simply lay one hand on her head or, if she will allow it, on her belly. Maintain a very light pressure so as not to interfere with any movements she needs to make – for some species of animal (particularly the larger ones) the process of birth can be a protracted one and involve lots of moving around and getting up and lying down. It is important to stay out of the way and let her get on comfortably and quietly. You should not intervene unless it is clear that she is

It is enchanting to watch a mother cat with her brood, cleaning, suckling and teaching her little ones, preparing them for the harsh world which awaits them. These few weeks of close contact between mother and offspring are vital, which is why the kittens should not be separated from their mother before a full eight weeks. By that time they will be independent and able to look after themselves.

struggling, and if so, telephone your vet for advice. If you are in a position where touching the infants is unavoidable, you can give healing to the young as they come into the world to provide a sense of comfort and peace rather than the usual shocking entry. However, your touch should remain as brief as possible and you should stay out of the way to allow the mother to birth naturally and bond with her young.

For the new mother, Bach Rescue Remedy can be given in water during and after birth to help to cope with the trauma, as well as Olive to help her to cope with general fatigue. You can continue to feed small amounts of Raspberry leaf to help the uterus to recover. To increase milk flow, you can add Cider Vinegar to the feed at the rate of one teaspoon per feed (if giving two feeds a day), along with herbs like Nettle, Fennel and Marshmallow.

Once the young start to explore and you are unlikely to disturb the ecology of the family unit by touching them, you can hold them gently for short periods and give them healing. This helps to strengthen young animals and provides a way to begin to bond with them. It can also give them confidence in being handled by humans. Try and let your young wean themselves as naturally as possible. Forced weaning is both unnecessary and unfair on mother and young. The young will begin to try their mother's solid food and steadily take less milk, at the same time becoming more independent. Make sure that, if you have to take the young away before they have become independent of each others' company, they have at least been introduced to the kind of diet they will be eating instead of their mother's milk.

A NATURAL WELCOME

If you become the proud owner of a young animal who has been taken out of the family unit, you are likely to suffer a few sleepless nights at first. Give healing treatments to help to settle a young animal and provide an environment of warmth, safety and calm. The best way to bond with your new pet is to gently hold him and give him energy as you get to know each other. Of course, this also helps in terms of physical health – the stresses of being taken away from mother and moving house can have a detrimental effect on young animals, who will generally respond by picking up every infection going. You can put a few drops of the Bach flower remedy Walnut into your pet's water to help him to cope with the challenges of change and adaptation to a new environment.

With a young animal, you will have to go through the fun of house-training (unless it is a small animal in its own cage or hutch, for example). With any animal, young or even adults from animal shelters, you will need to begin his education or reinforce the basic training, which will help you to get along with each other. For cats, there isn't too much of this other than learning his name, what he is or isn't allowed to eat and scratch on, learning to use a litter tray or go outside, and which exits he should and shouldn't use. For dogs, there is more to learn, with vital commands such as 'down', 'sit', 'lie-down' and 'stay', which help to establish some kind of order in the household and keep the animal safe in public. He may also have to learn when not to bark or jump at people.

Throughout any training process, bear your animal's needs in mind. For example, it's no good trying to teach your cat not to steal scraps if he's hungry and you feed him only once a day – he may need two or three small meals throughout a twenty-four-hour period. It's no good trying to house-train your dog if he needs to go outside every couple of hours and you tell him off for not being able to hang on while you're out at work all day.

This is not a manual on training, nor is it the place for lessons on how to teach your pet to do this or that, but remember that healing energy is an invaluable tool to help both you and your pet during the adjustment and learning process. Other pets within the family may need extra attention so they don't feel that the newcomer is getting all the fuss. Generally, it's a good idea to let animals work out who's who in their own way – after all, you can't keep an eye on every move they make, or be present at all times. Do supervise if it looks like one is in trouble, though, and use healing to help calm down all concerned and defuse the situation.

Animals who are newcomers to a household cope with their situation in different ways: some need a lot of fuss to make them feel secure; others prefer to withdraw and be left alone to settle in their own way. If you offer energy on a regular basis, your pet will know that you are available as a source of comfort and warmth and not just see you as the person who dishes up dinner. One thing that always interests me is how animals can recognize someone who practises healing. They gravitate towards him or her, particularly if they're tired or out of sorts. If faced with someone who doesn't work with energy when they've become used to having it on tap, they can get quite frustrated by hands that are 'firing blanks'!

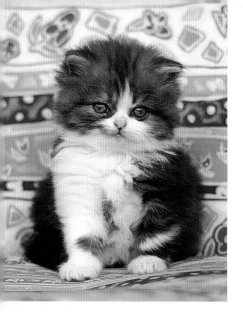

Be guided by your instinct and the animal's reaction, when choosing a new friend from an animal rescue centre. In the case of a puppy or a kitten, make sure it's lively and bright-eyed and do not separate it from its mother too early. Reputable animal shelters have visiting vets who make sure that the animals are in good health before being re-homed.

Opposite page. There are many dalmatians in need of rehoming. They are handsome, gentle dogs with boundless energy and a very active mind!

PICKING UP THE PIECES

If you're going to look for a new pet at an animal shelter, take your time, however difficult it may be. Resist all the pleading gazes of animals saying, 'Are you here for me?' In the same way as you wouldn't choose a human partner to live with just on the basis of the colour of their hair or shape of their body, it's crazy to choose a pet on looks alone. You need to spend some time getting to know each other, and often your instincts will tell you when you meet the right animal. Sometimes, it can be difficult to cope with an adult animal who may be traumatized, either purely through being re-homed or because it has had a questionable past, prior to coming into the shelter.

Not all animals in shelters have had a bad time: they're sometimes there because their owner died, suffered a broken relationship, moved abroad, changed jobs, had a baby or hit on hard times financially. Unfortunately, some rescued animals have had a really rough time and been deprived of food, company and the basic comforts. Whatever the situation, animals who have been through lots of change can find it difficult to settle and this, in turn, can be stressful for you. The more healing treatments you give them, the more you can help to rebalance them physically and release mental traumas. Reactions or habits that you don't understand can gradually be unravelled during treatments and it is at such times that you might be involved in an energetic exchange that helps you to understand how your pet feels or what he has been through. Of course, as you're getting a treatment at the same time, the more often you work together in this way, the better and more able to deal with things you will feel, too. Often people panic during the first few weeks of owning a new adult animal because they can't seem to get it together. As I always say, that creature has come into your life for a reason – the secret is to learn what the reason is.

People who have fostered children have told me that taking on a re-homed animal is a little like the fostering process. A lot of the reactive behaviour that children develop around the trauma of upheaval is the kind of instinctive behaviour that you see in animals. It seems that, deep down, we're all programmed to respond to stimuli from our environments on a very basic level. This is why I say that the more you study animal behaviour and apply that to people, the more you learn about human beings.

For example, one of the parallels I've learned about between re-homing both children and animals is that both can become very pushy and demanding of

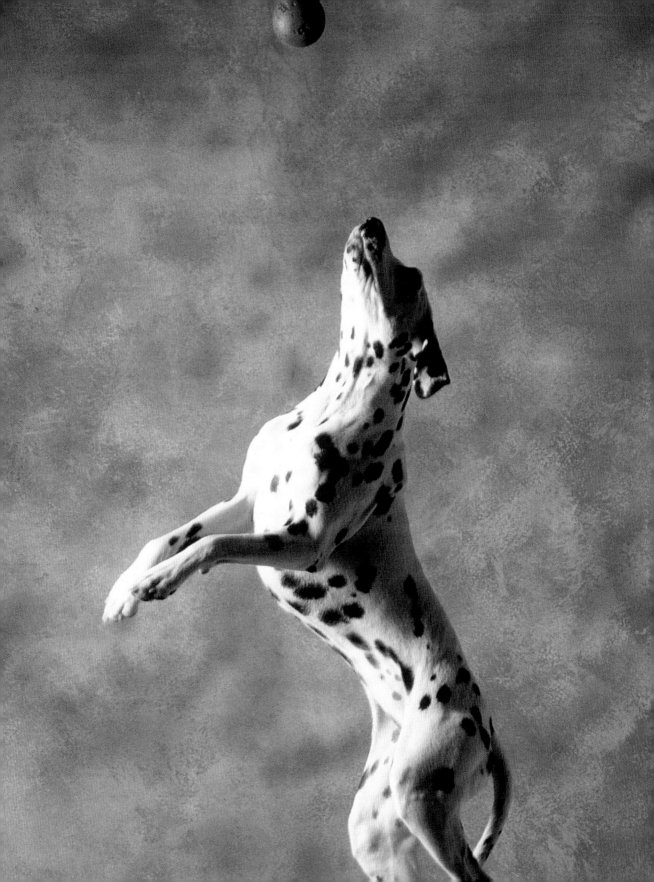

attention as they settle in to a new home. With time, this behaviour usually sorts itself out but, initially, it can be very trying. This process is one of establishing place and role – 'Who's the leader? Do I have to take control here, or will you protect me? Am I safe, or is there danger – if so, does the danger come from you or from a different source?' Cats tend to be a little shy and withdrawn about settling in to a new home, whereas dogs get out there and engage in the moment. Larger animals like horses, too, will go one way or the other and actively test the situation or totally withdraw from it. Remember not to over-humanize animals' behaviour and interpret what they do as personal – 'He just did that to annoy me!' You're likely to be projecting your feelings onto the animal – just because you're annoyed doesn't mean that your pet had any motivation for what he did other than simple curiosity, for example.

The settling process tends to take the form of a steady sequence of advance and retreat. To learn something, the animal will try something out. Then he'll assimilate what he learned from the experience. Of course, this is simply the model of learning in action. One way to make the settling and learning process a happy one is to use positive reinforcement at every step of the way – giving praise or reward for the desired or 'right' action, and ideally ignoring an undesired or 'wrong' action. Be fair and always consistent in your signals and try not to over-react. Animals can quickly become 'numbed' to owners who shout about everything and such de-sensitisation to your voice leaves you almost without any way of gaining your pet's attention. You can change tack and work a 'clicker' or other noise stimulus if you take on a pet who ignores voice commands. This is much less traumatic than using negative reinforcement, which, of course, works the opposite way. However, if necessary, and if you are careful, you can use negative reinforcement passively – an example of this might include putting something that tastes horrid on the furniture that you don't want your new puppy to chew. That way the negative aspect of the process doesn't come directly from you and you won't look like a tyrant!

Rewarding good behaviour with food can be counter-productive, though. Clever animals can quickly learn to respond only if you have a titbit to give them. It is far more sensible to use praise and a rub with healing energy as a reward. With some animals this becomes a motivation to learn in itself. Those who have been rewarded in this way often develop the habit of thrusting themselves into your hands for their 'blast', or even gently picking your hands up with their teeth or feet if you are slow to oblige! It is as well to make the learning process relaxed and enjoyable for both of you. Using healing energy as a reward certainly encourages this feeling but take care not to overdo it, or you may end up with a very bouncy animal or with both of you napping on the sofa – though what better way to end a training session?

The uses for healing energy in the ongoing process of getting to know each other are boundless, but on a deeper level, will provide a true sense of connection between you and the new member of your family. Be innovative and, should issues come up that result in difficulties with communication, keep working with energy to deal with the misunderstanding, blockage or behavioural difficulty that you experience. Rest assured that once you have begun to establish a bond, everything slowly slots into place. Most animals want nothing more than love and companionship from the humans they live with, so they prefer to make you happy; the same should go for the humans and their attitude to the animal.

LIVING ENERGY

Whether you are prompted to learn to work with energy as a result of reading this book, or whether you already work with some kind of energy therapy, it is true to say that it can completely change your life. People new to working with energy repeatedly report positive, sometimes dramatic changes of all kinds in their lives – from an improvement in physical health and emotional stability, to a complete turnaround in their way of living. They may handle stress and negativity better than before, and are also better equipped to understand what is important to their own happiness. Lots of people undertake a gradual clearing of the things that create difficulty in their lives.

Working with healing energy seems to improve your mental clarity, enabling you to focus on life in a new way. Your awareness of and sensitivity to the needs of animals and other people will be raised, and the benefits that you derive from this are countless. Working with energy can take as small or large a role in your life as you wish. For many people it becomes part of what they do, an extra dimension, which is always there in the background. For others, it becomes a whole way of life.

TREATING YOURSELF AND OTHERS

If you learn a healing art of any kind you will be taught to treat other people and, most probably, yourself. As you draw in energy it is passing through your body, so it will work on you as it travels. I sometimes wake up in the morning feeling less than enthusiastic, but after a couple of treatments I am totally recharged and raring to go. Many people find that the best time to treat their own body is at the beginning or end of the day, as part of their morning or evening routine. Treatment first thing in the morning can give you a wonderful sense of strength, clarity and peace with which to face the day. Last thing at night can be an equally good time to treat, and just resting a hand behind your head or on your stomach can relax you as you drift off to sleep, as well as recharging your batteries. It's also a great way to release the strains of the day and enable you to wake up feeling

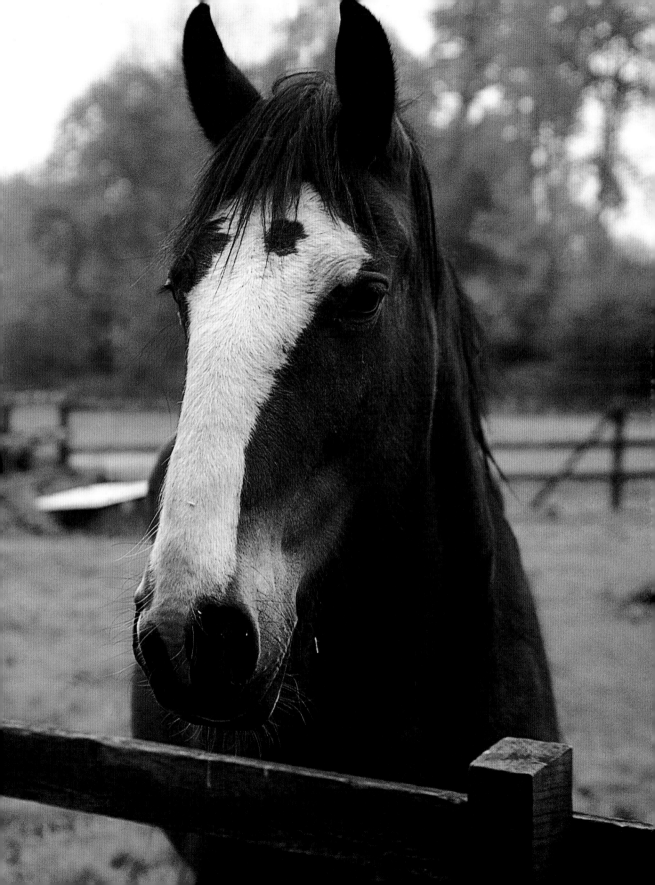

fresh and revitalized. For anyone who has difficulty sleeping, either with restless or broken sleep, treating yourself at night can help to induce a deep state of relaxation that carries you effortlessly through the night.

Because healing is the ultimate portable, silent therapy, you can also treat yourself whenever and wherever you want to, simply by placing a hand on your own body as you feel the need. I tend to 'plug in' one hand while I'm driving, sitting at my desk, even just resting a hand on my knee when I'm talking with a room full of people. If I'm walking around or standing, I sometimes plug a hand in to my hip to top myself up – nobody is any the wiser, though after a while people who know you will cotton on to what you're doing. As soon as you begin to feel tired, stressed or have a physical ache or pain of any kind, you can heal yourself to bring life back into balance.

One point to bear in mind is that because the energy has to pass through you, if you do have an imbalance or a need for treatment, this can reduce the energy that you project. This 'dip' in flow can even happen as you're giving a treatment – I have experienced it when bending over and treating someone in an uncomfortable position and I ended up with most of the energy going to my own back. Because the efficacy of what you're doing is running slightly lower than usual you may also find that treating others takes much longer or that they simply don't gain the full benefit of the work. If you find this happening, it is advisable to stop giving treatments for a while and work specifically on yourself until you feel the flow increasing in strength again. Your own need for treatment might be physical, emotional or anything in between, but focusing on yourself and giving yourself a treatment can help you to become aware of something that you have been putting to one side or haven't recognized.

The most effective way to establish a clear and strong flow is to use energy as much as possible; like flexing a muscle to strengthen it. If you consciously practise at first and begin to project energy whenever your hand touches your pet, yourself or a member of your family who enjoys treatments, it soon becomes second nature. A constantly available flow also keeps your own energy levels steadily recharged. Repeatedly drawing energy in is also the most beneficial way to maintain calm and the strength to deal with the 'stuff' that we all face in life: dealing with the bank, the washing-machine breaking down, going to the supermarket, getting stuck in traffic. It can also help you to stay level in difficult situations, like coping with your own emotional ups and downs. I always say to people that it helps you to wear the world a little more loosely. It is important to work on yourself to create a clearer path for the energy, and constantly using energy as you touch is a perfect way to achieve this. Treating other people is a natural spin-off from learning any healing art and is what many people start out doing. Usually you will begin by treating friends and family and progress to being asked to treat their friends and family as word spreads.

FINDING YOUR TEACHER

If you wish to go on to study healing formally you need to find someone who can help you. There are a few practitioners who specialize in healing animals and who teach others to do so. Generally, though, it will be easier to find a teacher of healing energy therapy who works with people, and then adapt what you learn for treating your pets. Once you have learned and can do it, it doesn't matter what kind of body you work on.

Your best option is the teacher who comes by personal recommendation – so ask around. The experience gained by others in learning from a teacher is worth far more than any advertisement. If you don't know anyone who is interested in healing, go to your nearest health-food store or 'new-age' shop – the kind selling crystals, self-help books and so on – who will have, if not resident teachers and practitioners, a list of contacts available locally. Pick up any magazine on complementary therapies or alternative healthcare and you will find advertised lists of courses, practitioners and workshops. Some doctors or vets may be able to tell you about therapists working locally, as may community centres and even churches. This area of work is thriving in terms of public interest so there will undoubtedly be someone not too far from you who will be able to help.

As the majority of people now have access to the internet, this is probably one of the first ports of call for anyone seeking information. You only have to key in the word 'healing' to any search engine to come up with a list of web sites on this and related topics. This is great if you're still at the research stage and haven't decided what you would like to learn. If you do know what kind of healing therapy you would like to study – so much the better. If there isn't a web site listed for anyone in your area, there are often umbrella sites hosting lists of practitioners and teachers. Failing that, contacting the people you do find can lead you to someone closer to home.

Opposite page. Cats are fascinated by anything which behaves like natural prey such as these floating leaves which move a little like mice.

Below. Pennyroyal (*Mentha pulegium*). This plant is a great natural air-freshener and deodoriser of pets' bedding. Orally it can be given in place of ordinary mint, though with care, as it is more pungent.

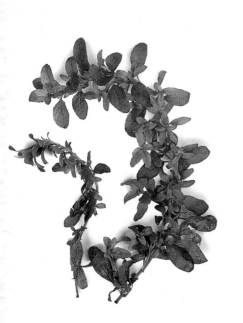

Finding a practitioner or teacher close to you is the first step. The most important part of the process is to make sure that you 'click'! You can work this out for yourself with a phone call, but if you're not sure, arrange to have a treatment for yourself (or your pet, if the person does work with animals) first, to see how well you get on. Do be aware, however, that there are therapists who don't teach. This may be because what they do is very individual and they haven't yet found a way to teach it to others, or because they haven't yet been trained to teach others themselves. There are a few people who are protective about their work and just won't teach – and are generally best avoided. They attempt to maintain an air of secrecy, mystique and power around working with energy. Needless to say, their attitude only serves to attract criticism to this kind of work.

Many teachers will have set dates for workshops but others will be flexible and agree to tutor a group of friends. Some will offer one-to-one training or will teach in pairs, while others will work in a group, which may be small and informal or on a larger scale. It is up to you to decide how you feel comfortable and how you will feel best placed to learn what is being offered to you. It's a once-in-a-lifetime experience, so decide how you're best going to enjoy it. It is also worth finding out about back-up for questions that may arise as you begin to work, or practical workshops that can help you as you develop your practice.

NUMBERS AND LETTERS

The basic energy that you learn to work with does not vary according to price! Learning to work with energy to heal should, in fact, be considered priceless – just as breathing or walking. The fee you pay is not for the energy itself – it's to cover the teacher's travelling, hire of the room, his or her time on the day itself and in preparation beforehand, as well as for catering and any teaching materials used.

Today there are many different kinds of healing energy therapy being taught, some of which have recognized 'qualifications', others are to set standards, and others still are unregulated. If you are learning a recognized healing art, your teacher will have been trained to a certain standard. With many energy therapies, the ability to pass energy on to others is not given until the final level of training. If formal qualifications are your aim, you will need to check that your teacher is qualified to train others. However, if gaining the ability to work with energy is your only real desire, you may find reputable teachers who will be able to offer guidance in their own form of healing practice which does not carry

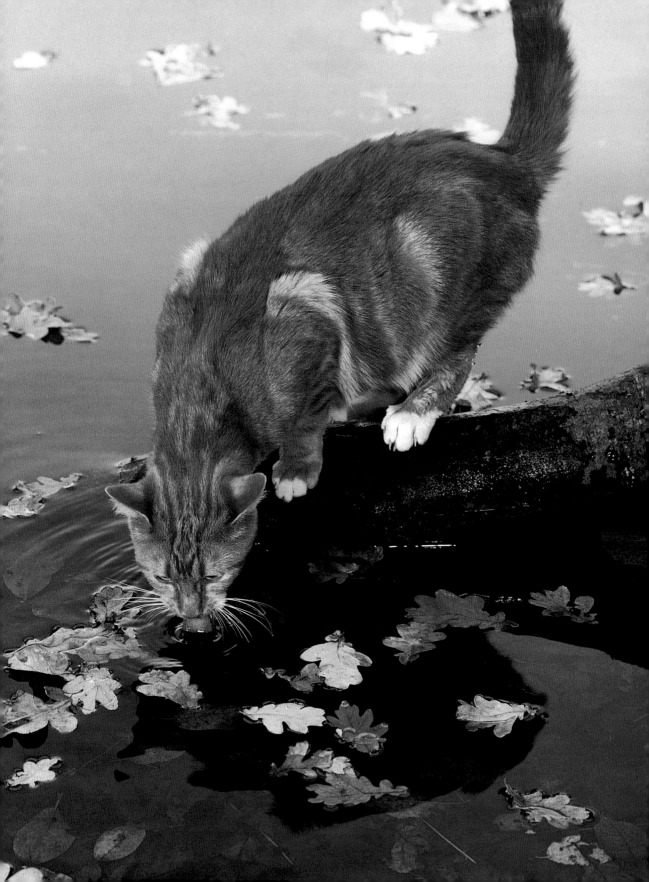

qualifications, letters after one's name and certificates. Many of the organizations which are perceived to be 'governing bodies' for a particular therapy are simply membership associations, so do check up what the letters mean if you are concerned. Remember also that all the qualifications in the world mean nothing compared with experience. I've met some wonderful teachers who were just little old guys that didn't even have a name for what they were doing. Your instinct will guide you as to a teacher's credentials – generally speaking, the individuals in this line of work are genuine people who want to help others. The charlatans aren't usually hard to spot.

WHAT WILL YOU LEARN?

The content of any training course will vary greatly according to the particular practice that you choose to follow. It is also true that teaching is very individual work and so personal style has a bearing on the material that each teacher conveys to his or her students. Even within practices, the methods of working and actual information passed on evolves from one generation of teachers to the next. The important point is that what you learn will be based upon the ability to draw in and project energy. Anything else that you are offered should be helpful and informative, but you will soon learn to take from it what you feel to be true to you.

Many energy therapies are taught in a split series of stages, and often over a given period of time to allow for practice and adjustment on the part of the student between each stage. It is entirely a matter of personal choice when and if you move on to each stage. Usually the main change at each level of training will be an increase in your personal energy levels, along with the energy that you are able to project. It is important that you undertake each stage of training as and when you feel ready and able to. Having your personal energy levels suddenly and significantly boosted can be difficult to handle if you aren't prepared for the next stage – sometimes it can be more difficult to handle for those around you!

Whatever kind of healing energy therapy you choose to learn, you are likely to find that, following initial training your own health will significantly improve. Students often go through some form of clearance, because starting to work with energy for the first time can be a fairly major healing process in itself. This clearance might be emotional or physical, depending on the 'stuff' that you have to shift. I always warn those who attend my workshops to expect something during the immediate week or so afterwards – they all nod and say yes, without really considering what their own clearances might involve. Because the nature of people who come to healing is so caring, often we are the ones who act as a shoulder for others to cry on. I have witnessed many memorable 'clearances' from students who are so caring to others that they have spent years denying their own feelings. These are the people who suddenly find that, as they clear and heal, all their buried feelings come flooding out – which can be pretty awesome. The whole point about this process is that it's positive, because it's about self-healing. It's difficult to work effectively to heal others if you're storing a lot of junk of your own, because the energy you draw in will be constantly working to heal you, and there won't be much left over to give your pet. Many people adapt quite naturally to the process, however, particularly those who have formerly been working with energy or who are undertaking training simply as a way to boost their own practice.

If you intend to treat people, check up on the law concerning human complementary practice; in the USA you should not touch the human spine unless qualified to do so. I always ask anyone with a hearing aid to remove it or turn it off during treatment in case the energy affects it in any way. For the same reason, I would not work on anyone with a pacemaker.

HEALING AS A WAY OF LIFE

If you do intend to work professionally with energy to help animals to heal, it is important that you gain experience before going out to work on other people's pets. One of the most rewarding aspects of working with animals is witnessing their recovery and their owners' happiness. There is something very special about seeing someone smile out of sheer delight and being there as part of the process. If you have recently started giving healing or have worked on humans before but not on animals, the basis of your work should be the same as it is with people – offering treatment compassionately and unconditionally, with your best intent.

People who hear that you work on animals will often ask you to treat their own pets. This can be how healing animals can become a full-time job, particularly if you love the work. Legally, you should have insurance that covers you to work on someone else's animals, and make sure that the pet owner is aware that he or she should tell the vet that you're treating the animal. Most vets are fine about animals having healing because it's non-invasive and can't do any harm. It can also help to enhance the effects of any orthodox treatments the animal is having and can be used alongside any other complementary therapy.

It's amazing how word spreads when people hear about what you're doing, and word of mouth is the highest recommendation there is. Just doing what you do without making a song and dance about it, even if your intention is only to treat your own pets, your family and yourself, can bring all kinds of people and animals to your door. Lots of people are just curious to begin with but soon get hooked on having treatments as a healthy, relaxing treat for themselves and their animals. Sometimes it takes a few curious people, or someone who has an animal that really needs help, to give you the confidence to work on subjects other than your own pets. If you ever find yourself lacking confidence and

My young horse, Daws Ace of Hearts, Here Ace is about two years old, and was regarded as 'potty' because of his behaviour in the field. Regular sessions of energy healing taught him to approach people and gently ask to be touched.

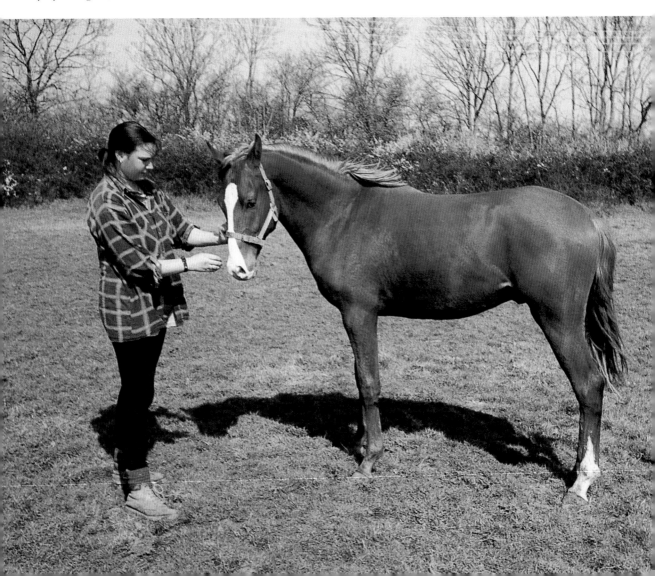

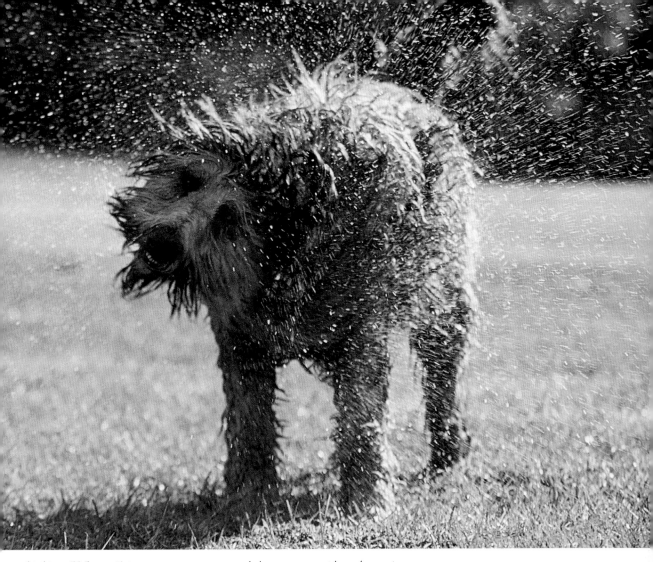

thinking, 'Why me?', just put your own mental chatter to one side and trust in the energy to do whatever the individual needs it to do. Remember, it's not you doing the healing and the results aren't down to you, so just relax and let it happen. You get what comes simply because you're the right person to handle it.

For example, I never 'set out' or 'decided' to become an energy therapist/healer, it just happened because that's what I'm here for. Sometimes, I'm faced with a dangerous animal, a person I'm not sure how to handle or a request to do something I'm uncertain about. When I feel my conscious, human mind creeping in with an element of doubt, I merely continue with whatever comes up and wait to see what happens. Situations like these are a way of learning a new lesson and the best thing to tell yourself is that 'everything is happening as it should'. If you simply allow life to happen and follow the path of least resistance, you develop a sense of detached curiosity, delight and understanding on an almost moment-to-moment basis. It is thrilling to see the sheer synchronicity of events as they unfold around you. Life is a journey, so go with it, explore it and enjoy the experience. The best way to enjoy it is to look at every new shift as an exciting development – an unrepeatable, unique experience that will enrich and enhance your own process. If you approach your work with an open heart and mind, all kinds of directions unfold that you would never have thought likely or possible.

If you want to make healing your work, the best way to start gaining experience is to offer treatments for free, or a reduced fee, until you feel confident and experienced enough to build your own practice. I often have students who come to me for training saying that they want to work with animals because they're happier around them than they are with people. Well, with this work, you get both. If you're not good with people, necessity teaches you to be more at ease and to approach each new person or animal you meet as an individual that you have plenty in common with.

This work also places you in a role where you have to find a way of mediating between the needs or agenda of the animal and those of the people involved. Often, this means that the people caring for the animal you're treating need to make changes or adjust their own beliefs. It's not always easy to play the middle-man, but experience will show you how to handle different situations as they arise. Sometimes, I go out to treat a dog and end up working on the whole family. In stressful circumstances, treating the people around the animal you're working on can help, and sometimes I feel that the animal is flag-waving on behalf of his owners. There are also situations where people project their own feelings onto their pets – in other words, they'll call you out to deal with a sick cat, when they are the one who needs healing.

Some of you will learn or have learned healing in addition to other therapies. Healing combines well with massage and other forms of bodywork, including aromatherapy, reflexology, shiatsu and acupressure. Each of these therapies can be used on animals, especially the larger ones such as horses. Some people combine aromatherapy, shiatsu and healing, for example, to form an integrated therapy. Acupuncture is another treatment where the practitioner's energy is involved, and healing can provide a potent addition to the use of needles. I have also trained people from the medical community who like to offer healing as part of their work, whether in a veterinary hospital or a human one. Medical staff involved in first aid and accidental trauma situations report that giving healing as they work helps to calm and relax the patient, which is invaluable during an emergency situation. Children respond particularly quickly to healing, which will soothe and calm them when they're hurt or frightened.

Because healing and orthodox medical approaches work so well in combination, it makes sense to develop a relationship with the professionals that you may encounter in the course of your work – vets, doctors and any other therapists involved in the care of the animals or the people you treat. Some of the medical profession can have a negative reaction to complementary therapies. It's important to impress upon people in this position that what you're doing is totally harmless and could be highly beneficial to their patient. If you can't be allies, it's as well just to do what you do quietly and without upsetting any applecarts – just 'leaving the door open'. Sometimes this allows people to go away, think about it and come back in their own time to approach you in a way they feel comfortable.

DISTANT HEALING

Some forms of healing teach you to 'send' healing remotely, or from a distance. Making a connection with another individual from a long way away is primarily about tuning into their energies – the energetic frequencies of other souls. The distance doesn't have to be vast – you can use distant healing from across the room, which is really helpful if an animal is frightened, stressed or aggressive. For people and animals who aren't nearby, you can learn to send energy using a photograph of the subject you want to heal; in time, as you become more sensitive to tuning in, you are unlikely to need one. It does help to have met the subject first but you may find you can simply 'pick them up'. I usually ask for a name and age and then visualize the animal or person receiving energy. When you send healing to animals, it can be a good idea to set a time with the owner so that, for example, you're not trying to send energy as the dog is going for a walk, or as the horse is about to be ridden. Animals can doze off just as effectively when they're getting a distant treatment, so scheduling is a good idea.

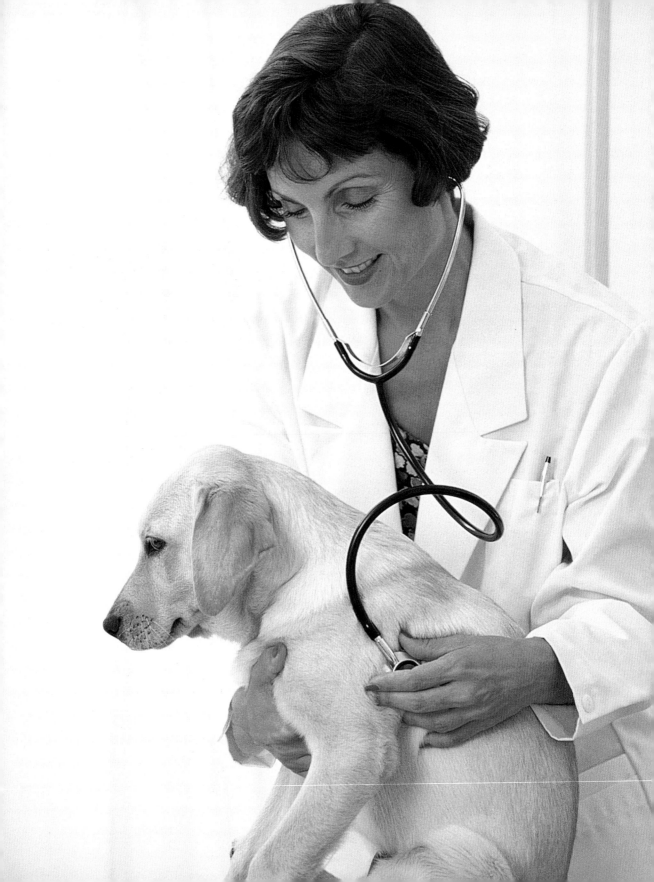

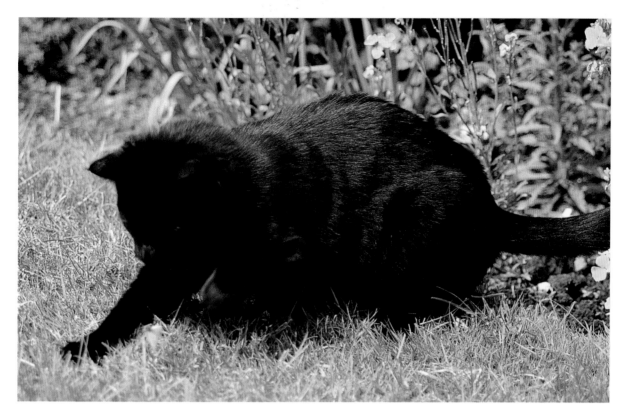

This kind of work is immensely valuable whenever you can't be nearby. People from the opposite side of the globe can ring and ask for healing for their cat, horse or family member (I regularly send healing to a cat in Washington, USA). If you know other people who work with energy, a powerful way to help a person or animal who needs healing is to ask your friends to send energy to the same individual; that way they receive the combined treatment of many people. It's a little like the idea of praying for someone who's ill; the intent of many people all wishing one individual well has a strength of its own.

The concept of healing from a distance is something that prompts lots of people to think about doing it 'on the sly'. Just recently someone rang me and asked me to send healing to his son, and commented how ideal it was that I could send him healing from a distance because he would never be open to it if he knew. I found this amusing but had to explain that if an individual doesn't want healing, he or she will simply block it. With distance work, that's fine because you can just send it to the earth or someone nearby who needs the energy instead, which you can also do if the individual you're sending it to has had enough or doesn't need it.

Above. Cat hunting in the grass. With distant healing, you can treat your cat as he plays.

Opposite. More and more vets are becoming sympathetic to the use of complementary therapies in the treatment of animals. It makes sense to develop a relationship with the vets in charge of the animals you may also be treating. It is important to emphasize that what you do is harmless and could be highly beneficial to their patients. Some vets employ nurses trained in energy therapy, or learn it themselves.

TEACHING OTHER PEOPLE

There is something unexpectedly delightful about getting out of life what you put in; an energetic form of karma. A great way to contribute to the lives of other animals and people is to teach them to work with energy for themselves. In time, you find that the intent with which you undertake to teach other people returns to you in the form of yet more wonderful experiences. Teaching other people is incredibly rewarding in so many ways and to anyone asked to teach others, I wholeheartedly recommend you do it. The process of unfolding realization is remarkable to witness each time and everyone brings their own unique approach to a workshop. When I'm teaching I feel privileged and humbled to be invited into the lives of so many other people and animals, and each new situation is a delight.

There's something really wonderful about the smile that springs to the face of anyone whose hands 'work' for the first time – children and adults alike. People I have helped to teach have gone on to do the most incredible work and to touch so many lives in countless special ways. They often tell me about the experiences they've had in the course of their work and I feel that my own role is very dull in comparison. Helping other people to learn is an immensely rewarding process. I find that, when I start each day, aside from a loose plan in my head of what I would like to pass on, I never know what's going to transpire. This is one of those situations where guidance from whatever higher source you believe in just takes over. The energy created where groups of people with a common intent come together can be startling, too, so workshops always turn out to be excellent fun and really uplifting. Sometimes at the end of the day I reflect on how incredibly lucky I am to be part of this process, to meet so many positive, giving people and to enjoy such a fascinating and delightful life. All of this sounds rather honeyed but it's true. If your focused intent is to help others on their path, the help which returns to accompany you on your own path literally seems to be multiplied.

SUPERVISION

Whether you simply treat your own pets, or whether you work full-time treating other animals or people, you need supervision. This is basically about having someone to talk to and share your experiences with – the age-old idea of 'healer, heal thyself'. Ideally, you need someone who will provide you with back-

Opposite page: Bonding with a new pet is all about finding common ground. Games with a stick are fun for puppies and people alike, especially with such an enchanting canine friend.

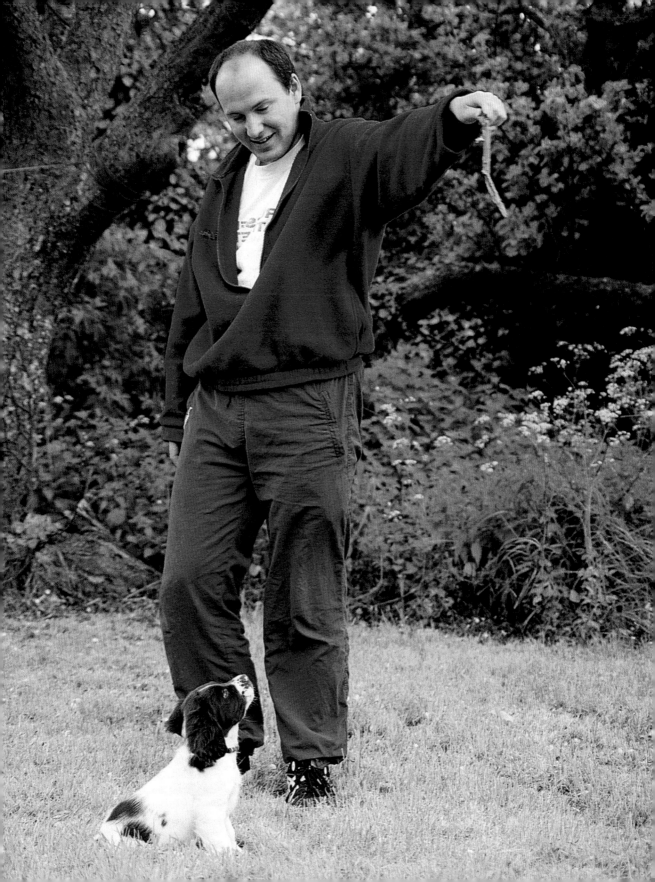

up, and occasional guidance as you work. Lots of people who learn to work with energy from a teacher will go to that person for supervision for the sake of tapping the insight that comes with experience. Sometimes, you may just come across the right person or discover that a friend provides the sounding board or backup that you need. The important part is that you should feel completely comfortable with the individual and that you can share literally anything with him or her. People who work in isolation lack a yardstick for their experiences: they don't know whether what happens is 'normal', or they get stuck trying to make sense of something that happens. In such cases it helps to compare notes with others who may have experienced something similar.

Supervision provides the opportunity to 'ground' what you experience – to bring it down to earth and to lighten the load. It's a good way to make sure that you don't carry with you what you don't need mentally, to shift the clutter so that you can be fresh and clear for the next treatment, the next animal or the next person. Otherwise, you can end up not dealing effectively with what you're doing because you're taking on and holding some of the negativity you encounter. This hardly leaves you in a position to bring health and happiness to others. I always say it's a bit like trying to throw someone over your shoulder and attempting to carry him when your own leg is broken. Sometimes people who work with energy get the idea that, with such incredible resources on tap, they can cope with everything. This is basically missing the point about healing – if you keep taking things on and don't let them go, you'll simply end up getting sick as well.

There is also a myth that people offering healing should be perfect, whole and hundred percent healed themselves. The fact is, if any of us were that perfect, we simply wouldn't be here! We're all human beings who continue to live and grow. A little turbulence shows that you're still alive, so engage in and learn from it, instead of sweeping your own worries under the carpet.

People who work with the same kind of therapy often take an opportunity to meet and share their experiences with each other. It's great to spend time with like-minded people who will make sense of what you say. Giving treatments in pairs or groups is a powerful process which enables you to share what you have learned individually. It's also enjoyable to have a treatment to help clear any personal issues, or just enjoy a little pampering. One thing that therapists of all kinds tend to suffer from is the 'bussman's holiday' syndrome, i.e. they don't

'Giving treatment in pairs or groups is a powerful process which enables you to share what you have learned individually.'

treat themselves because it's just like work! Sharing treatments can offer a way to remember how valuable a little time out for yourself can be, enable you to recharge your batteries and be more effective in your dealings with others. It's all very well taking on the world's problems on your shoulders, but make sure you are in top condition to cope with them..

Once you begin to work with energy, a whole new way of living opens up. You can learn about and experience life in a completely different way and form a deep connection between yourself and other animals. For anyone who simply wants to understand their own animals a little better, or to help maintain their health and wellbeing, the way to do so is here and now. The future is in your hands – so what are you waiting for?

'Once you begin to work with energy, a whole new way of living opens up.'

... AND FINALLY

My aim in writing this book and in all of the work that I do is to bring healing back to where it belongs – to everybody. The man in the street can be made to feel a long way removed from things so-called complementary or new age, and that shouldn't be the case. The message I hope to convey is that there's nothing new or strange about any of this; it's as natural as breathing, as natural as life itself, because it *is* life itself. Yes, there can be and, there often is a lot of play and show around something like healing, but don't let that bother you. This won't last much longer, because a climate in which everyone can learn the same skill is a great leveller.

I'm told that I have a very down-to-earth approach to something as esoteric as healing. That's exactly as it should be. Bringing a little touch of something from 'out there' down to earth can only benefit the people and animals it reaches. Helping people to make contact on a common level with animals serves to reveal a little of the mystery behind what we experience and perceive. In turn, this can help to improve the lives of so many people and animals, each of whom touch the lives of others. In the long term the greater benefits will spread to our environment and way of living among each other.

All I ask that you learn from this book is what feels true to you. To most of you, I suspect that the idea that you can heal with energy but can't quite remember how, feels right, deep down. Let your animals teach you what you need to learn – they can even help you to meet the people who will enable you to find what you're looking for. As you learn, apply your insight to the people who live around you. Remain open to new input and aware of how energy permeates your world: from the way you feel, to the health of your pets, the words and phrases you use, the way in which other people behave and how everything, ultimately, fits together.

One important lesson we can learn from our animals is about behaviour and communication. Communication and behaviour as an expression of energy are crucial to learning to understand other people. Next time you meet someone and think, 'he's got a chip on his shoulder', think for a moment about that

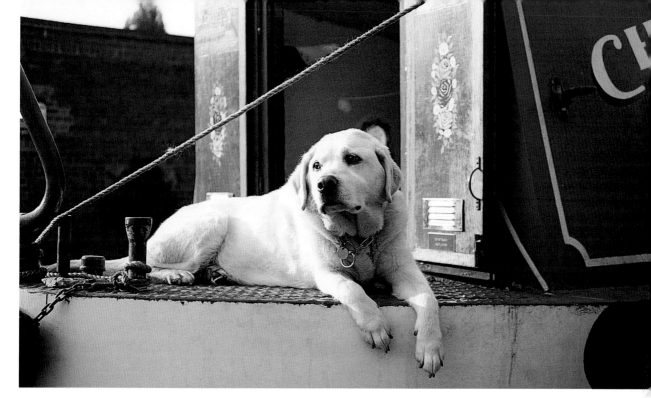

individual's experiences and perceptions of the world, and his reactions in terms of physical health and behaviour. Have a look at his shoulders, for a start. The sounds and movements that we make with our bodies as a result of what we perceive have a very raw, very basic, power. Tracing the origins of words that you use without even noticing, or habits which you've never even questioned, is an enlightening process. People are beginning to realize that, if they can worry themselves sick, they can also think themselves well – it's all about energy.

A 'down-to-earth' approach is, I believe, one of the ways in which the gap between orthodox and complementary practices can be bridged. Ultimately we're all people who care and we all want to help ease suffering, particularly where animals are concerned. I believe we all have a responsibility to work together for the greater good. Vets are becoming much more open to complementary work, so always 'leave the door open' – it's surprising who comes back to find out a little more. There are now vets and veterinary nurses who themselves trained in energy therapy, while many other vets' practices will refer patients to healers in the way that the human medical community does. I know that the animals will appreciate it, and it's one small way of reducing the 'us and them' attitude that permeates so much of society. 'Us and them' is only ever constructive if it's taken as a starting point to work towards 'us' – towards

Under the right circumstances, pets who are happy to be with you can make ideal travelling companions. Dogs in particular, usually greatly enjoy the experience.

unity. I would also like to see healing and other complementary work become specifically available and accessible to people who own animals. Everyone should be aware of what they can do to help care for their animals themselves, so that the days of struggling to find someone who can help are over.

Whatever you take from this book and however you choose to work with energy, remember that the animals in your life led you on the way. I'm not sure who it was that decided we humans aren't animals. I'm not sure why people think they're somehow 'better' or 'more civilized' than the other species we share the earth with. It's an outdated view and one that, as everything does in time, calls for review. Healing is all about compassion, and compassion isn't species-specific.

On an energetic level, we're all pretty much the same anyway; we're all just souls in bodies doing what we're here to do. Learning to heal our animals is the first step to understanding how we all fit in to the world together and how each of us can benefit the lives of other species of animal, as they, in turn benefit us. The story of Scoot, outlined below, is a testimony to the greater understanding which healing energy can bring between animal and owners.

To anyone taking their first steps towards working with energy, I would like to offer a few very simple thoughts. Just let what happens happen, in the knowledge that you're learning what you need to learn. Live every single moment because the journey you're travelling, the life you're experiencing, is so very precious. Opening up to energy is opening up to the richness, magic and the simple wonder of life – the path that you tread will amaze and delight you.

Scoot steps out

At seventeen years old, Scoot has seen a lot. He's a Thoroughbred, owned by Michaela and her fifteen-year-old daughter, Amber. He stands at 15.3 hands.

Scoot always did very well at shows and behaved perfectly when being ridden, but he could be difficult to handle on the ground, particularly in the stable. He threatened to bite, could be difficult to catch and refused to stand still while being fitted with new shoes. He had always behaved like this and it seemed to stem from the time when he had lived in a big yard with some seventy horses, competing every week, never leaving the stable and without any real companionship – a real workhorse. Because he was such a gentleman to ride, Michaela and Amber, in particular, wanted to get to the bottom of his problems and try to help him be a happier horse.

Scoot hadn't worn back shoes for several years. He had suffered a bad experience with a farrier who, startled by a nearby horse kicking out, had accidentally hit a nail into a sensitive part of one of Scoot's hind feet. Scoot had panicked, tried to get away, broken his lead rope and charged around, all the time treading the nail further into his foot. He ended up sliding over on the concrete yard and had to be sedated by the vet so that the farrier could get the shoe off again.

Michaela and Amber brought Scoot to stay on my yard for a month, in the hope that I could help him to relax enough to have his hind feet shod. It was a tall order in just a few weeks, and I suggested that at least one of them should learn to work with energy so that they could carry on with the treatment at home. The first thing I noticed about Scoot was that his musculature was unevenly developed through his shoulders and back – he was quite 'one-sided' and his saddle wasn't helping him very much. As I began treating him it was clear that although he had some habits that were difficult to cope with, they did not stem from anger or pain, but were part of a mechanism Scoot had developed as a way to cope in his earlier life.

I worked on Scoot three days a week and he began to settle down – I never had a problem catching him and any 'faces' he made in the stable seemed to be a half-hearted attempt that he forgot about by week two. I was concerned that his body be helped to heal so that he would be more comfortable, as this would clearly have some bearing on how easy he was to catch and handle generally. I also worked on him with my own farrier to show him that there was nothing to fear. The farrier had a good look at Scoot's feet and said, 'You know, his feet are really hard. He seems to have adapted to working without hind shoes on. He doesn't honestly need them.'

Amber came to a training workshop to learn to use energy, and did her first practical session on Scoot. She knew almost nothing about healing before she came and was amazed to find that her hands 'worked' by the end of the day!

We continued to work on Scoot but, by the end of the third week, it was clear that it was going to be a very, very long job to get him to the point where he would trust a man with a hammer and nails near his hind feet again. I felt that, for the horse's sake, it was kinder to stop trying to acclimatize him to something he really didn't need anyway and I explained this to Michaela and Amber when they came to fetch Scoot. They took him home, surprised to learn that he didn't need the shoes they had been trying so hard to get him to accept, and decided to adapt their own ideas, and to leave him without hind shoes. After all, he was sound and always worked well, so they were happy to let him go on without the unnecessary trauma.

A month later, his owner got in touch to let me know that she had continued treating Scoot three times a week. They had bought a new, much wider saddle, which had already helped him to develop his muscles more evenly. Amber was surprised that, as his shape improved and he clearly felt more comfortable, he became easy to catch and far more at ease in the stable – no more biting or snapping. An unexpected bonus was that Scoot seemed to have far more energy, was moving freely, and his stride had lengthened and become more bouncy – all due to his new shape and saddle. He was stepping out so well that she had taken him to a local dressage competition and come second two days before, winning him a smart new saddlecloth.

Matty's bad day

Matty is a four-year-old yellow Labrador bitch who accidentally got herself into a spot of bother. Her companion, a terrier named Penny, had a habit of disappearing down rabbit and fox holes. One day, in the thrill of the chase, Matty started to squeeze down inside a hole after Penny and very quickly got badly stuck. Penny, meantime, had a great fight with a fox and made a hasty exit from the hole she was in with some fast and furious digging – and Matty stayed stuck. Their owner eventually managed to loosen enough of the earth to get Matty out who was by then, quite lame in her front legs. The vet's examinations showed that she had damaged the muscles around her shoulders as well as some of the ligaments in her legs; the damage meant that she would have to stay indoors for several weeks to recover before she would begin to walk normally again.

Matty's owner had learned healing and used it regularly to maintain her horse's health and wellbeing. She treated the dog's sore muscles and ligaments twice every day, for ten or fifteen minute-sessions. One week later, Matty was sound and happy again. She hasn't looked back since. She certainly no longer follows Penny down holes!

The space and freedom to roam is important to cats who like to have their own 'patch' where they can escape and observe the world from.

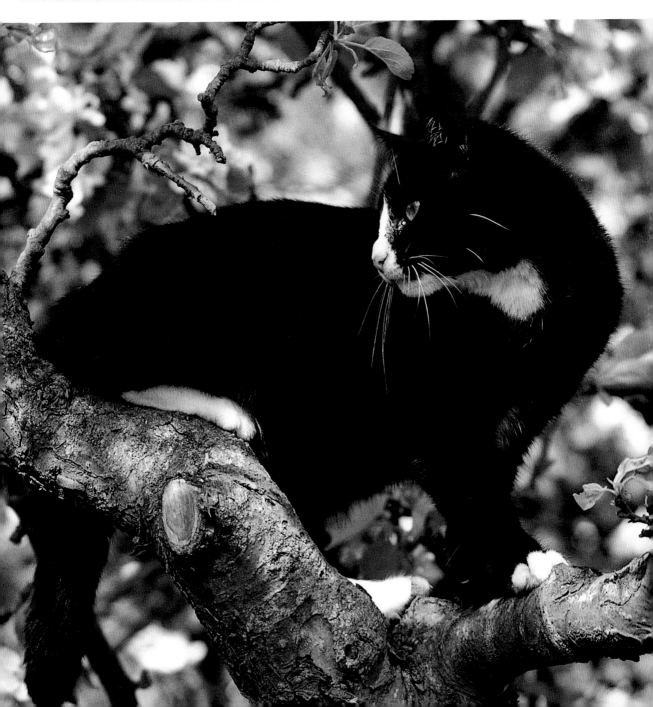

Misha's story

Priscilla came to one of my healing workshops with her boyfriend, Keith, because she was interested in finding a way to relieve her own chronic back pain. Following a car accident some four years ago, Priscilla, a thirty-six-year-old teacher, had undergone a number of operations to her legs and spine but remained unable to walk or stand for long periods, experimenting debilitating pain in her back. As she could no longer exercise her profession, Priscilla's time was now spent gardening and breeding Burmese cats.

Her family of cats is headed by Misha, a beautiful female, now in her fifth year, who has produced two litters of enchanting kittens. Having learned to use healing for herself, Priscilla found that the often aloof and very private Misha suddenly became far more attentive and demanding of her company. She could clearly sense the change in Priscilla's energy and loved nothing better than to spend hours close to her owner in the garden. Misha simply 'asked' for her blast of healing by coming and sitting on Priscilla's gardening tools or gloves, as if to request a 'time-out'.

Surprised and delighted at the remarkable shift in her cat's attitude, Priscilla decided to pursue her healing training to the level where she could help to 'attune' others to the energy. I told her that I often attune animals when I treat them. So that they can draw in as much energy as they need to, which is helpful in times of sickness or stress. Fascinated at the prospect, Priscilla decided to see if Misha would like an attunement as she was gently treating her on a particular evening. Misha loved the energy and rolled over to play, patting Priscilla's hands as she worked with her. Later that week, Priscilla rang me: 'I don't believe what is happening with Misha,' she said, 'now when I work on her, it's as if she's giving me energy back, too!' She explained that she could feel the warmth of the energy, right down through her legs and feet as Misha sat on her lap for her own treatment. It's true that our animals have a particular 'knowing' about much of what we discover. Yet Priscilla certainly hadn't expected her cat to be a natural healer, working with energy to help her in return.

APPENDIX

FREQUENTLY ASKED QUESTIONS

Who can learn healing?

Anyone.

Do I need to prepare, or have any qualifications to learn to heal?

No. You don't have to be gifted, spiritually inclined, believe in anything in particular or understand how it works. You don't even have to believe in healing for it to work. You don't need to prepare or do anything special to learn to heal. All you need is an open heart and mind and a willingness to help others.

Do you get tired?

No. That's a myth. The only time people get tired when they're healing is if they're using their own energy. If you use the energy that is available all around you, you actually get the benefit of it as it passes through and so you feel energized and stronger after working with it.

Do you take on the condition of the body you're working on, feel their pain or get sick?

No. Your own energy is at such a level as you're working that you don't succumb to negativity. You can't pick up the illness or condition you're treating. You may be aware of the individual you're working on experiencing pain or discomfort as this is reflected in their energy, but you don't feel it yourself.

Could I do anything wrong?

Not if you just offer healing for the individual's benefit, without involving your own agenda. You can't do harm, hurt anything or open any 'cans of worms' because the body you're working on dictates the treatment. Always treat injuries from the sides of the area and make sure that first-aid or appropriate attention is given where indicated.

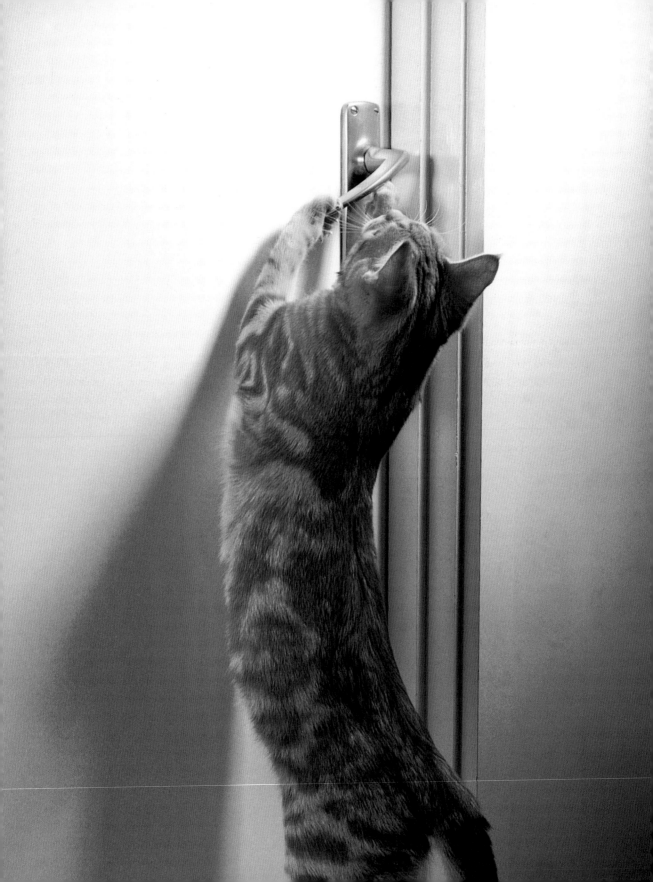

Are some forms of healing more powerful than others?

The outcome of any healing is not down to the practitioner, but is entirely dependent on the individuals being treated and how they react to the energy. In this respect it's impossible to measure if one practice is in itself more effective than another.

What will I learn if I go to someone for training?

This varies entirely according to the particular healing art you decide to learn. The content of your training is likely to include some background and theory on working with energy, attunement to the energy itself and practical work.

How much training must I do before I can offer healing to other people's animals?

You can offer healing with very little formal training, because you can do no harm with energy. So long as people are aware that you're not a medical practitioner, you can work as a healing therapist.

What else should I study that might be of help?

There are many courses available in all kinds of complementary therapies that may deepen your understanding of energy in its healing capacity. However, there is no substitute for experience and the more you work with energy, the more you will learn from it.

Opposite page. And we think they need us! This cat has obviously worked out a few things in the confusing and unnatural world in which he lives.

INDEX

ACKNOWLEDGEMENTS

Photographic credits:

The photographs on the pages mentioned are reproduced by the kind permission of their copyright holders: page 7: Jane Burton/Bruce Coleman Collection; p 11: John Hickman; p 18: Julie Meech; p 19: Telegraph Colour Library; p 27 (top): Brian Hoffman, Telegraph Colour Library (bottom); p 30: Julie Meech; p 31 (top): Andrew Cowin; p 42: Brian Gibbs; p 50 (top): Andrew Cowin, Paul Beard (bottom); p 51: Barbara Marshall; p 54 (top): Brian Hoffman, Brian Gibbs (bottom); p 58: Jorg & Petra Wegner/Bruce Coleman Collection; p 59: Barbara Marshall; pp 63 & 75: Brian Gibbs; p 79 (top): Holt/Nigel Cattlin; p 82 (top): Holt/Jean Hall; p 98: Telegraph Colour Library; p 99: Hans Reinhard/Bruce Coleman Collection; p 102: Telegraph Colour Library; p 103: Brian Gibbs; p 111: Julie Meech; p 115: John Hickman; p 118: Nick Board; p 123: Jane Burton/Bruce Coleman Collection; p 126: Andrew Cowin; p 127: Telegraph Colour Library; p 131: Nick Board; p 135: Kim Taylor/Bruce Coleman Collection; pp 139 & 142: Telegraph Colour Library; p 143: Brian Gibbs; p 145: Nick Board; pp 149 & 153: Julie Meech; p 156: Jane Burton/Bruce ColemanCollection.

Special photography: Pages 2, 10, 15, 22, 23, 31 (bottom), 35, 39, 43, 46 (top), 67, 70, 78, 79 (bottom), 82 (bottom), 83, 87, 91, 114, 134: Curtis Lane & Company; pp 46 (bottom), 47, 71, 74, 94, 107: Trevor Meeks.

Pages 122 & 138: supplied by author.

A special word of thanks to:

ARC – The Animal Rescue Charity, Foxdells Lane, Rye Street, Bishops Stortford, Herts CM23 2JG.
(Registered charity, donations always welcome!)

Hingston Farms Bed & Breakfast, Piggotts Mill, Thaxted, Essex. Recommended accommodations for those attending healing training workshops in Thaxted.